Rudraksh Therapy

*Ancient Herbal Healing Miracles
Rediscovered for the Holistic Health,
Mental Peace and Life Prosperity of Mankind*

*A Comprehensive Scientific Exposition of the
mystical & medicinal potentials of the
Indian Herbal Bead - Rudraksh
(Elaeocarpus ganitrus)*

Professor B.D. Sharma
Ph.D., D.Sc., Gold Medalist, SMN (UK)

DIAMOND BOOKS

Publisher : **Diamond Pocket Books (P) Ltd.**
X-30, Okhla Industrial Area, Phase-II
New Delhi-110020
Phone : 011-40712200
E-mail : wecare@diamondbooks.in
Website : www.diamondbooks.in
Edition : 2025

Rudraksh Therapy
By: Professor B.D. Sharma

Acknowledgement

The author is deeply indebted to
his wife, Dr. Tej Kumari,
son Vikram Devakar and
Daughter Dr. Vandna Sharma
for their moral support and
consistent encouragement
during the completion of this book.

Preface

The inception of integral relationship of the holy bead of herbal RUDRAKSH for the well-being of mankind is as old as human civilization. The origin of herbal healing system of rudraksha therapy dates back to the Vedic period of India.

A review of nearly 5000 years old available ancient Indian literature evidently reveals that mankind had always deep reverence for the HERBAL HOLY BEAD OF RUDRAKSH. Several references are on record i.e. related to the effective usage of the *mystic, religious, spiritual* and *medicinal potentials of rudraksh.* Since several centuries the people in India and in particular of the neighbouring countries in general have widely practised the holistic healing and spiritual efficacy and medicinal values of rudraksh.

The rapid strides of recent researches have also confirmed the scientific validity of the preventive and the curative potentials of rudraksh for the well-being of health and life prosperity of mankind.

In Ayurveda, which is the ancient medical science of India, the rudraksh has been referred as the king of all *Herbal Medicines.* The immense importance of rudraksh, therefore, necessitates its extensive cultivation in all agro-climatically suitable regions of India.

Since 1970, the author has been making several experiential and experimental observations on rudraksh therapy. The innovative researches of the author based on relentless perseverance were thematically aimed to develop the rudraksh therapy in a perfect way. My studies also endorse that the therapeutic use of rudraksh is not only effectively preventive but it also cures all energy disharmonies in the subtle energetic spectrum of "*Body-Mind-Soul*" complex in terms of the unified nature of bio-energy field.

As an economic, harmless and restorative healing system the rudraksh can best be called as: - A NATURAL AND PERFECT HEALTHCARE SYSTEM or HOLISTIC REMEDIAL SYSTEM OF THE TRADITIONAL AND COMPLEMENTARY MEDICINE.

The present book aims to contribute up-to-date and comprehensive studies on the herbal healing miracles of rudraksh. The book contains bio-ecology of rudraksh together with its mystical and medicinal potentials. Thematically, the book compounds the experimental and experiential knowledge of the author with the overview of contributions so far made on rudraksh Therapy.

Hopefully, the book which as a rare and unmatched contribution on the subject is first of its kind. It will serve indeed as a valuable source book for all the natural and herbal health conscious people in general and the rudraksh therapy practitioners in particular.

The author would welcome suggestions from the entire spectrum of readership of this book so as to enable him to incorporate the necessary updates in the subsequent edition.

Prof. B.D. Sharma
D.Sc.

Founder : Holistic Rudraksh Therapy
Research Foundation International,
Life Fellow Herbal Academy, USA
Life Fellow Rudraksh Academy International
Scientific Advisor to CRIMS - Govt. of India
Natural Excellence Award in Rudraksh Therapy

Founder: **Holistic Healing Foundation International**
P.O. Box 3, Gandhi Nagar, Jammu (J&K) 180004 India
and
Dr. Vandna Sharma
(Physician Consultant)

Contents

Section I : INTRODUCING RUDRAKSH

Section-II: IMPORTANCE OF RUDRAKSH

Section III: RUDRAKSH THERAPY FOR PRACTICE, RESEARCH AND DEVELOPMENT

Contributors

1. Professor G.S. Lavekar

   Director
   Central Council for Research in
   Ayurveda of Sidha (CSRAS)
   No. 61-65 Institutional Area
   D-Block, Janakpuri, New Delhi-110058

2. Dr. Sunil Sobti

   Mahek Info Arts Pvt. Ltd.
   B-57 Vivek Vihar
   Phase-II, Delhi-110095

3. Tanay Seetha and Kapil Khanna

   63, Aram Nagar-1st Seven Bungalows,
   Andheri (West)
   Mumbai-40006 Maharashtra

4. Ms. Neeta and Dharam Deva Arya

   G-1, Ekta Society
   Near Worli Bus Depo
   Next to Vithul Mandir
   Sasmira Marg, Worli
   Mumbai-400030

Section I

INTRODUCING RUDRAKSH

Chapter I

Rudraksh: An introduction & scientific description

What is Rudraksh? : The Definition

The holy bead of rudraksh is dried herbal nut stone (endocarp) of the fruit of rudraksh tree. The seeds are carried inside this bead. In English vernacular the tree of rudraksh is also called *blue marble tree.* The bead of rudraksh is, therefore, nothing but the innermost stony part (endocarp) of the fruit of rudraksh tree.

Legendary perspective

The etymology of the word rudraksh reveals its age-old linkage with the Sanskrit scripture of India. It owes its origin from two root words viz. **Rudra** means Lord Shiva and **Aksha** means eyes. This denotes the meaning of rudraksh as 'eye of Lord Shiva.'

In Rigveda, *Rudra* is the original name of Lord Shiva. There are several legends about the origin of rudraksh on earth but all ultimately pertains to the relationship of Rudraksh to the eyes of Lord Shiva. Due to the age old divine legend associated with the origin of rudraksh it is deeply rooted in the religious and spiritual dimensions of Hinduism.

According to one of the most popular ancient legends, there was a powerful demon named "*Tripurasura*" who used to fight the divine holy men (*Devtas*) and kill them mercilessly. Lord Shiva, the supreme power of the universe, was greatly displeased with this demon (*Tripurasura*) due to his sinful actions. Hence, Lord Shiva decided to kill 'Tripurasura' by using a powerful divine weapon "*Manohara Aghora*". After killing the demon, Lord Shiva was so much delighted that the tear of joy started rolling from His eyes. These tears which fell on earth, became holy beads of rudraksh enthused with mystical, spiritual and medicinal properties.

The Vedic scripture of India also describes that the holy bead of rudraksh contains the secret of entire cosmic evolution. The study of Indian mythology is as old as entire cosmos or universe astoundingly reveals that several species of rudraksh which existed on earth long ago are still growing without any fast extinction of its species during the long course of history of evolution.

One of the remarkable features of rudraksh tree is its ability to withstand the rigors drastic evolutionary changes which could modify or wipe out the species. The origin of rudraksh species took place in the time immemorial era which sprawled many years before the origin of dinosaurs, snakes and other giant creatures which ruled over the earth.

All these huge and horrible creatures lived for several million years and disappeared for ever due to hectic rigors of climate & of calamaties. It is indeed astonishing that the rudraksh species are still continuing exercise; they are grown in the nature of Himalayas.

Family of Rudraksh

Plant and Species

In botanical terminology, the genus of Rudraksh is known as ELAEOCARPUS.

(Elaeo = oil, Carpus = fruit).

Hence the name has been given to it due to its fruit which contains oil.

Species: The plant of rudraksh belongs to the floral family: **Elaeocarpaceae:** A review of the world literature reveals that as many as 360 species under twelve *genera* in this family of rudraksh are known from world over (Tiral 1982 and Lee 1998).

Remarkably, the family of rudraksh which is known by 360 species has worldwide distribution. The genus of rudraksh is *Elaeocarpus* which is represented by over 30 species in the world of which 25 have been reported from South Asia. Some common species recorded from India are described as under:

(1) *Elaeocarpus ganitrus*
(2) *E. sphaericus*
(3) *E. grandis*

(4) *E. floribundus*
(5) *E. oblongatus*
(6) *E. pertiolatus*
(7) *E. serratus*
(8) *E. tuberculatus*

Tiral (1982) has synonymised *Elaeocarpus ganitrus Roxb* and *E. sphaericus* (Gaertn) under one species only, viz *Elaeocarpus angustifolicus*.

General Geographical Distribution of Rudraksh

The berry of rudraksh was first spotted in Indonesia. Ecologically, the species of rudraksh are widely distributed from Nepal to the Himalayan foothills to the South East Asia, China, Sri Lanka, Bali, Indonesia, Java, Jakarta, pacific Islands, Sumatra, New Guinea to north Australia, and even Hawaii.

Nepal is believed to be the original birth place of all rudraksh species. It is the only country which produces maximum cultivation of rudraksh in its Bhojpur area Dhingla in the Arun Valley of Nepal, famous for large and excellent varieties of rudraksh.

Nepal also specializes in producing the best quality of rudraksh of high export value.

Java is the only country which produces not only the largest size of rudraksh bu t also the streakless variety of rudraksh bead which has no vertically grooved lines on it.

Such types of natural and specialized rudraksh beads are known for their largest size without vertical grooves on them which are exported from Java to various parts of the world. These varieties are also called 'zero faced' rudrakshs. Some of these large grooveless rudrakshs have no roughage due to absence of protuberances on the surface. Hence, their surface is flat & they are named as AMLASAR RUDRAKSH. Studies have revealed that this type of rudraksh is very effective in the cure of cancer.

Some Indian Species of Rudraksh with Distribution and Local Names

As many as 28 species of rudraksh have been reported from India under the single genus: ELAEOCARPUS.

Distribution in India: Rudraksh is widely distributed in India in evergreen forests which are moist, deciduous and located between altitudes of 1500 m – 2000 m. It has been reported to grow in Bihar, West Bengal, Sikkim, Assam, Arunachal Pradesh, Meghalaya, Nagaland, Manipur, Mizoram, Tripura, Orissa, Maharastra, Andhra Pradesh, Karnataka, Tamil Nadu, Kerala and Andaman & Nicobar Islands.

In its eco-Geographical range, rudraksh is distributed in Sri Lanka, Bhutan, Bangladesh, Myamar, Indo-China, China, Malaysia and Indonesia.

Distribution of Some Common Species with their vernacular names in various regions of India is as under:

1. *Elaeocarpus tectorius* (Lour)

Region	Local name
Assam:	Poreng, Selong
Garo Hills:	Agong, Bolrongong
Kanada:	Hinnalatorde
Malayanam:	Kattu Kara, Malam kara
Orissa:	Nard, Champa, Panasia, Patragundi
Tamil Nadu:	Bikki

2. *Elaeocarpus tuberculatus Roxb* (Deccan Olive)

Region	Local Name
Kanada:	Bhuttali, Dandemora
Malayanam:	Pilahi Naggara Rudrak
Tamil Nadu:	Rutthra cham

Distribution in India

This species thrives well in the moist evergreen forests located between altitudes of 1500 m - 2000 m. It has been reported from Bihar, West Bengal (Darjeeling) Sikkim, Arunachal Pradesh, Meghalaya (Assam), Nagaland, Manipur and Maharastra.

Extra-limital Distribution

Beyond India, it is reported from Nepal, Bangladesh, Mayanmar and Malaya.

3. ***Elaeocarpus stapfianus*, Gagnepain**

Region	Local Name
Arunachal Pradesh	Seleng

Distribution in India: It is widely distributed in Arunachal Pradesh in the evergreen forests located between 800 m and 1000 m.

4. *Elaeocarpus sikkimensis*

(Hindi = Bhadraksh)

Region	Local Name
Assam	Seleng
Indo-Nepal	Bhadrase & Nepal

Distribution in India: It is found in West Bengal (Darjeeling), Sikkim, and Meghalaya (Assam). This species thrives in the semi-evergreen forests located between 1500 – 2000 m.

Extra-limital Distribution: Bhutan

5. ***Elaeocarpus ganitrus*** **Roxb**

= E. Sphaericus, (Gaertn)

(Utrasum Bead tree or Wooden Beggar Bead Tree
In Sanskrit = Rudraksh.)

It is the most common species of Rudraksh in India.

Region	Local Name
Meghalaya (Assam):	Rudrai
Telugu:	Rudrakshalu Rudraksha
Tamil Nadu:	Akkam, Rudrakai Rudraksha
Orissa:	Rudrakhyo
Bengal:	Rudraksh; Rudrakhya
Gujarat:	Rudraki
Malayanam:	Rudraksha
Kanada:	Rudraksha

Distribution in India: It has been found to be the most common species with wide distribution. The natural population of this species is abundantly found in Bihar, Bengal, Madhya Pradesh, and some parts of Mumbai. It is also occasionally cultivated as ornamental plant.

General Description of commonest Rudraksh Species

Elaeocarpus ganitrus Roxb.

(Blue Marble Tree)

Habitat Altitude: 700 – 1700 m

Tree Size: The tree is large & evergreen. It is as big as banyan tree & takes 15-20 years to grow. In usual height, the tree grows to 25 feet with girth of 3 feet.

Bark : The bark of rudraksh tree is dark, rough and marked with small scales.

Leaves: The leaves are oblong oval in shape. The size varies from 3" to 6". Each leaf has a highly toothed leaf edges.

Flowers: The flowers of rudraksh are creamy and most attractive in look. The blooming takes place during rainy season and flowering during March-May. The flowers are bisexual (hermaphrodite) and are born in cluster. The inflorescence is axillary raceme type. The flowers arise mostly from the axils of old leaves.

Fruits (Drupe): The fruit of rudraksh is one of the most brilliantly looking fruits of the world. The creamy celute flowers give rise to green fruits which first turn purple and then brilliantly blue when fully ripened. It is globose or 0.5 – 1.0 mm in diameter. The fruiting (fruitfication) takes place during October-December. After removal of the outer skin (exocarp) the upper part of the fruit is light brown and pulpy. The bluish purple fruit is highly nutritides & slightly sour in taste. The fully ripened fruit is frequently eaten by birds and animals. It generally encloses a 5-celled stone or bead.

In shape, the fruit of rudraksh is globosal and varies in size from 0.5 – 1.0 inch in diameter. It contains hard innermost nut or fruit stone (endocarp) hence, called drupe or berry.

Bead (Endocarp): The holy bead of rudraksh (Fig. 1) is nothing but the fruitstone enclosed within the pulp of the fruit. It contains several seeds encapsulated into it. It is about the shape of a berry with size variation from 3 mm to 40 mm.

Each rudraksh bead has hard texture with a central continuous aperture. The roughage of surface is due to several uneven protuberances which are natural formations in a genuine rudraksh.

In addition to several protuberances on a rudraksh, there are longitudinal furrows on it which are also called facets or mukhs. Based on the number of these facets, the religio-spiritual classification has been done for various significant uses of these varieties.

Normally, only one specific facial variety is found on one tree only. Hence, for every facial type of rudraksh, the tree is different.

The beads of rudraksh are of high economic value. These beads are cleaned, polished and sometimes stained for making rosaries, bracelets and other ornamental items.

As many as 3000 rudrakshs can be collected from a single tree. Of this huge production from a single tree, 20% production is inferior, 60% is average and the 20% is the best.

The harvesting for holy beads of rudraksh is done every 2 to 4 months before maturity of beads.

Seeds: Each bead of rudraksh contains 4-5 black coloured elongated seeds. Different species of rudraksh produce differently coloured seeds which are potential source of medicinal oil.

The matured seeds remain viable for 2-3 months. However, the viability can be extended upto one year at lower temperature. The natural germination of seeds without any treatment of fertilizers etc. is 20% to 30%. The original seeds of rudraksh also never float on water unlike spurious ones.

Wood: The wood of rudraksh is very hard and known for its remarkable strength ratio to weight ratio. It is highly valuable timber.

During the period of the First World War, the wood of rudraksh tree was extensively used in the making of propellers of the aeroplanes.

Chapter 2

Physical Characteristics of Rudraksh Bead

Physical Structure (Morphology):

The holy bead of rudraksh is a hard nut (endocarp), round to oval in shape and hollow from inside in which it carries seeds. It has a natural hole (central canal) in it from one end to another.

The upper end (anterior end) of every rudraksh bead has a small epical cone. It is also called face end or *Rudra/Shiva*. However, the lower or basal end (posterior end) is flat and without a cone. It is also called the pedicellar end or naval end – *Brahma*. In between upper and lower end, the bulged body is called *Vishnu* end.

The surface of each rudraksh has several ridges (protuberances or tubercles) which provide roughage to it. *No two rudrakshs have similar type of protuberances like the 'finger prints' which are never alike in any two humans.* This wide variation in finger prints is unique and remarkable in rudraksh. In addition to such ridges there are deep clear longitudinal furrows visible as vertical lines each starting from the pedicellar end (flat or lower end).

The deep longitudinal furrows divide the inner hollow space of the rudraksh bead into number of compartments which contains seeds. Normally, 4-5 seeds are found in a bead.

Shape Varieties of Rudraksh

With regard to shape, all available species of rudraksh are known to exist in the following shapes and forms. These shape varieties have been discussed in detail in the science of Ayurveda–

1. Round shape (*Rudraksh*)
2. Oval or flat like almond. It is half moon shaped that's why it is called *Ardh-chandrika* (*Kaju Dana* or *Badam shape*).
3. Long – semi round shaped (Rondraksha).
4. Sadraksh (Subhaksha).

Size: In size, the rudraksh is known to be found as small as black pepper and as large as Ambla (*Emblica officinalis*) or table tennis ball. It varies from 0.25 to 2 cm. According to Meru Tantra, the bigger size of rudraksh and Shiv Linga are effective for prayer. The hard, big and highly ornamented rudraksh are considered virtuous in effectivity. The smaller rudraksh beads are highly valued as rosary as they are easy to carry and wear.

Colour Varieties

There is a wide diversity in the colour and shape of rudraksh. It is a universal fact that no two rudrakshs have exactly the similar shape and colouration. There are four main colour varieties of rudraksh which are commonly available:-

1. White colour rudraksh
2. Honey Colour rudraksh
3. Black colour rudraksh
4. Mixed colour rudraksh

Classified Facial Types of Rudraksh

Based on the number of furrows following facial varieties (mukhis) of rudraksh are as follows:

No. of furrows	Facial type
1. One furrow	(Param-Brahama/Shiva
2. Two furrows	(Shiv-Shakti/Shiva Parvati)
3. Three furrows	(Tridev-Brahama, Vishnu, Mahesh).
4. Four furrows	(Chaturanand/Brahm Swaroop).
5. Five furrows	(Panchamukhi/Rudranga (or) Kalyani Swaroop)
6. Six furrows	(Shiva Putra/Lord Kartikeya).
7. Seven furrows	(Sapta Matrika/Sapta Rishi)
8. Eight furrows	(Ganesh/Vatuk Bhairav).
9. Nine furrows	(Nav Durga/Dharam Raj)
10. Ten furrows	(Dash Avtar/Janardhan).

11. Eleven furrows (Indra).
12. Twelve furrows (Vishnu-Shiva).
13. Thirteen furrows (Vishvedev).
14. Fourteen furrows (Bhuneshwar/Hanuman)
15. Fifteen furrows (Rudhra, Divine Gem or Devmani)
16. Sixteen furrows (Pashupati Rudraksh)
17. Seventeen furrows (Vishwakarma Rudraksh)
18. Eighteen furrows (Bhumi Rudraksh)
19. Nineteen furrows (Nargana Rudraksh)
20. Twenty furrows (Brahma Rudraksh)
21. Twenty one furrows ((Kuber Rudraksh) or Laxmi Rudraksh

Some aberrant shape varieties of rudraksh of high spiritual significance:-

(1) A Doublet Rudraksh (Gouri-Shankar)

It is symbolic to Lord Shiva and his wife Parvati. Hence it contains the power of Shiv-Shakti. It is a single compound rudraksh in which two rudraksh beads are jointed at the head end. Such a form is rarely available in nature. As a religious-spiritual remedy, by wearing this doublet rudraksh the relationship between husband and wife becomes more attractive and life-long. It is also known to enhance the fame and wealth resources. For maximum benefit of wealth, it should not be worn but kept in the Cash Box/Money Box or safe to fulfill the aspiration of wealth.

(2) A Triplet Rudraksh: (Triguni or Trijugi)

It is highly speicialized form of rudraksh which is also known as Brahma – Vishnu – Mahesh swaroop. It is known to represent three supreme divine powers (Gods as per Hinduism) which balance the cosmic energy cycle of this universe i.e. cycle of life & death in the process of evolution of all life forms. It also enhances the intuition for inventing new researches.

Three most powerful divine powers represented by this rudraksh are cited as under:-

1. *Lord Brahma* – Creater – Brings about evolution of bio-energy in all living forms (*Cladogenesis*)
2. *Lord Vishnu* – Sustainer – Brings about sustenance of all life forms (*Stasigenesis*)
3. *Lord Maheshwara* – Destroyer – Destroys and transforms the life forms and energy cycles (*Anagenesis*).

(3) Gauri Path Rudraksh

In shape this rudraksh is round to oval in shape with two laterally raised ridges parallel to each other. It is considered best for unmarried persons who do not get suitable match for marriage settlement.

(4) Ganesh Mukhi Rudraksh

This holy bead of rudraksh has a typical lateral protrusion like the belly of trunk of the lord Ganesh. It is used to enhance the wisdom of prosperity.

(5) Nag Rudraksh (Snake shaped rudraksh)

This rudraksh looks like a sitting snake (Nag). It is essentially a rudraksh which is known for its rare of the rarest status in availability. It is essentially for keeping in your prayers and not for wearing. It wards off the fear of snakes and enhances the prosperity of life & harmony in the family by removing all negativity. The Kal Sarp Yog of a person as per astrology can be effectively cured if he keeps a Nag rudraksh in his pooja sathal (Prayer room).

Classification based on faces of rudraksh (faces of rudraksh classified)

A genuine rudraksh bead is always known for its clear and continuous longitudinal furrows on the surface.

Based on the number of these longitudinal furrows so-called faces, the rudraksh has been classified from one to twenty one faces. However, there are references of rudraksh upto 38 faces (Mukhi) in the ancient Indian scriptures of Puranas.

Till date we have now one to fourteen mukhi of rudraksh available and the rest forms are uncommon or rare. One faced rudraksh is very rare. Two and seven are easily available whereas 8-14 facial varieties are uncommon and 14 to 21 faced rudraksh are also rare in their status of availability. The main causes of fast depletion of the valuable varieties of rudraksh include it's over commercial exploitation and ruthless destruction of its natural habitats. Indeed, if it could go unchecked more varieties of the previous heritage of our rudraksh flora would doom to extinction or extermination.

All what we need today to save rudraksh species is to undertake extensive cultivation, scientific farming and establish *gene pool banks* for future research and development studies on rudraksh.

Chapter 3

Test for Genuine Rudraksh

Identification & Quality Test for Rudraksh

It is essential to know the authentic identification of genuine rudraksh before using it as any spiritual or therapeutic remedy.

(I) Best Quality

The best quality of rudraksh is known for the following salient features.

(1) It is always good looking and shiny sublime in texture.

(2) It has always the brightness of its natural colouration. Honey colour (i.e. dark reddish brown copper colour) is considered to be the best. However, the pinkish coloured rudraksh is best for medicinal use.
Other good rudrakshs are also found in various shades & colouration viz., whitish, black, yellow, reddish & even mixed colouration.

(3) The vertical streaks (facets) on the best quality of rudraksh are sharply defined (deep) and evenly distributed (unbroken).

(4) The central hole of a genuine rudraksh is natural, continuous with unbroken margin (rim).

(II) Better Quality

The better quality of rudraksh is known for the following characteristics which are as under:

(1) The texture is not much shiny, smooth & comparatively less attractive.

(2) The colouration is light in shade. Generally, it is of clay shade.

(3) Some verticle lines (longitudinal facets) may not be even in distribution.

(4) The central hole which is natural may not have the even (unbroken) rim.

(III) Good quality

The rudraksh of this quality is known for the following characteristics:

1. The texture has a very little shine or glow.
2. The roughage of the texture has irregular distribution of protuberances.
3. The colouration is generally light brown or lightest brown. Generally, 2 streaked (two mukhi) rudraksh belong to this group.
4. Most of the streaks on the surface are not sharply deep.

(IV) Bad Quality

The quality of rudraksh is considered to be bad due to following characteristics:

(1) Dull in look with uneven roughage due to tubercles of uneven size & irregular distribution on the surface.

(2) Dented, broken, unshaped (defaced), insect eaten are always considered as bad samples.

(3) Discontinuous vertical streaks and also the broken rim of the central hole degrade the quality of rudraksh.

Tests for Genuine Quality of Rudraksh

In order to rule out the maximum possibility of its being fake the purchase of rudraksh should always be through a genuine seller.

A rudraksh bead is tested for its genuine quality by using various prevalent methods described as under:

1. **Water Dip Test:** Take a glass of ordinary water & dip the rudraksh into it to observe as under:
   (1) If it drowns (sinks) it is genuine.
   (2) If it floats, it is fake & just a wooden dupe with lighter density.
   (3) If it just submerges, it is genuine but not fully matured (ripened) naturally. However, older genuine rudrakshs also loose their sinking capacity. Hence this test is not so authentic for the genuine & quality grade best rudrakshs.
2. **Boiling Water Test:** Put the rudraksh in boiling water for five minutes to observe as under:
   (1) If its fissures (vertical facets) are not damaged, it is genuine.

(2) However, if the fissures break or disappear, it is not genuine.

3. **Milk Dip Test:** It's one of the oldest and known methods. Just dip rudraksh in the pure unboiled milk of cow in which no water has been added. A genuine rudraksh will float whereas fake will sink.
4. **Milk Test:** Keep the rudraksh in milk (boiled or unboiled) & observe as under:

   (1) If the milk is not spoiled for a longer period than the normal time, it indicates that the rudraksh is genuine.

   (2) If it gets spoiled just sometimes after contamination which indicates that the rudraksh is fake in quality.
5. **Copper Plates Test or Magnetic Polarity Test:** Keep the rudraksh vertically in between two copper plates or coins and gently press the plates.

   (1) If it slightly moves (rotates) due to electromagnetic effect of polarity, it is genuine.

   (2) If it does not show any movement, it is fake.

It's not so positive or authentic test because any round thing placed as such can show polarity dynamics.

6. **Black Stone Test:** The black stone called "Kasoti" which is commonly used by the jewellers for testing the carat value of gold, can also be used for testing a genuine rudraksh.

   Just rub the rudraksh on black stone & observe as under:

   (1) If an impression is made on the stone, it is genuine rudraksh.

   (2) If the impression is made on the black stone, the rudraksh is of fake quality.
7. **Presence of Seeds Test:** A genuine rudraksh bead will always have black oblong seeds located in various compartments inside it.

   (1) The presence of these seeds can be heard by jingling it swiftly near your ears. But it is a difficult exercise & does not give assured results, because the jingling sounds of the seeds is very mild & low.

   (2) However, when broken a genuine rudraksh bead will show the presence of seeds inside located compartment.

How to Preserve and Enhance the Maturity of a Genuine Rudraksh to Harness Maximum Benefit of Effectivity?

A rudraksh removed from a fully rippened fruit is, fully matured, natural & gives maximum benefits.

All samples of rudraksh which are collected from their trees are not fully matured (ripened).

Most of the beads are generally immatured (unripened) in which even the seeds are not fully formed. It is just because of the over-commercial exploitation of rudraksh. This is to get quick and enormous commercial gains. Most of the immatured beads which are collected from their fruits can be easily diagnosed due to their aberrant physical features.

In any case, if a rudraksh bead is matured or immatured it has to be duly preserved for its longevity & effectivity of potentials.

The preservation of rudraksh beads can be done by the following methods:

Before using rudraksh samples (single or many), they should be immersed & soaked in pure mustard oil for about seven days. Take out these oil soaked rudrakshs from the mustard oil & wipe out with cotton or cotton cloth the excessively smeared oil traces from the surface of each rudraksh. Remaining traces of oil associated with the surface of rudraksh can be removed by giving 1-2 washes in soapy water and a final wash with ordinary water.

Now such oil soaked rudrakshs can be dried up with a cloth & even in open sunlight. This method of soaking in oil preserves the longevity and healing potentials of rudraksh. However, it preserves the rudraksh getting damaged from the insects. It also protects the rudraksh from excessive heat & extremes of temperature effects which cause cracks and crevices.

Section II

IMPORTANCE OF RUDRAKSH

Chapter-4

Cultural, Religious, Spiritual and Commercial Importance of Rudraksh

Cultural Importance

The cultural importance of rudraksh is deeply rooted in the religious & spiritual heritage of India, Nepal in particular and South Asian countries.

Throughout in India and south-east Asia, the rudraksh is used as religious or social jewellery. The holy beads of rudraksh are reputed as most beautiful ornamented berries of the world. In various cultures of Nepal & south-east Himalayan regions, the people use rudraksh as '*sacred ornament*' in the form of necklaces, bracelets, arm-amulets, ear-rings & even fore-head jewellery so much so that various decorative items are made from rudraksh & given importance as cultural & religious sanctity in houses.

The rudraksh made items are not only considered auspicious and sacred but also best for the restoration of health, wealth, mental peace & well being of mankind.

Religious Importance

Religious association of rudraksh is an integral part of Hindu culture & in particular Shaivism. Rudraksh plants are considered to be the most sacred plants by the Hindus.

Rich & varied diversity of religious rituals of the Himalayan regions of India & Nepal attach more significance to the use of rudraksh. Hindu mythology acclaims highest reverence of the holy beads of rudraksh & its potentials for the cure of all ills & evils & also for the empowerment of spiritual energy.

In Hinduism, the rudraksh is worshipped as a true embodiment of "Lord Shiva". The Hindus refer rudraksh as eye of Lord Shiva (*Rudra*: an epithet of Lord Shiva and *Akshya* means eye) It is considered to be the best spiritual tool for blissful meditation & prayer.

The ritual use of rudraksh is also considered to expand the consciousness & awaken the serpent power (Kundalini energy).

The holy ash of rudraksh called *bhasm* or *vibhuti* are a trident of rudraksh known as that the *trishul* has highest sacred status in Shaivism in particular and Hinduism.

According to "*Padam Puran*", the holy beads of rudraksh are widely recommended for all denominations of human society, irrespective of caste, creed and religion. Even an atheist and sinner can get equal benefit by wearing the holy beads of rudraksh. Taking bath in rudraksh water is considered as sacred as a bath in the water of the holy Ganga River.

It is due to the immense socio-religious protection and reverence to rudraksh by all the people in its ecological habitats that various species of rudraksh have survived even today. These surviving species have successfully faced all relentless crises caused by men & nature during the course of long history of evolutionary period. Even today, the population of rudraksh plants are always protected, preserved and revered by men as the most significant forest resource.

Spiritual Importance

Rudraksh has always been realized as spiritual medicament in India, Nepal & many south-eastern countries. The saints, seers and spiritual seekers have always revered the spiritual potentials of rudraksh far awakening & empowerment of spiritual energy potentials for them.

Rudraksh is also used as a powerful "talismic tool" with dynamic supernatural & divine potentials for the cure of all ills & evils.

Late Mrs. India Gandhi Ex-Prime Minister of India always used to wear *Ek Mukhi* (one faceted) rosary of rudraksh. She always attached much spiritual significance to it. No other rosary or holy bead is as powerful & auspicious as rudraksh.

Likewise, Yehudi Menuhin, BKS Iyenger and several other top brasses always used rudraksh rosary with great spiritual reverence.

The spiritual use of rudraksh has been enormously highlighted in 'Shaivism" as '*quintessential regalia*'. It is known to ward off or neutralize all negative vibrations of planetary or human origin (enmity, evil effects etc.)

Economic and Commercial Importance

Since centuries, the rudraksh has been used by mankind to get a wide range of benefits from it. The multifold benefits of rudraksh with its mystical, religious, spiritual & medicinal potentials have always augmented the demand for genuine rudraksh both in National & International market. Such a prolific use of rudraksh by the mankind has added to its commercial importance.

Various uses of rudraksh in relation to its economic & commercial importance are as under:

(1) Rudraksh as currency

In the countries like Nepal, rudraksh is being used as currency. The best quality of rudraksh beads has always accelerated its demand. For instance, one mukhi rudraksh which is known for a single longitudinal natural groove on it is highly prized for its potentials of blessing, spiritual bliss and holistic prosperity.

One best quality of single facial rudraksh may cost even one lakh rupees. Another equally prized rudraksh is zero facial which has no longitudinal grave on it.

(2) Rudraksh as spiritual Remedy

With the advent of new era of researches in consciousness studies and spiritual sciences, the demand for using rudraksh has also been greatly amplified. Rudraksh is now being frequently used as a remedy for spiritual healing, spiritual and energy empowerment, blissful meditation. In contact therapy rudraksh is potentially effective spiritual healing herb when used as a rosary or single bead pendant.

(3) Rudraksh for meditation and Kundalini Power

.Rudraksh is very helpful in spiritual exercises of quick & blissful meditation, Kundalini awakening (serpent power). These exercises are essentially for restoration of inner peace & spiritual empowerment.

(4) Rudraksh in Astrology & occult sciences

Rudraksh is invariably used as an astrological remedy and also as an effective tool in the accomplishment of several occult exercises like sidhis, supernatural powers and advanced tantra.

Ancient Vedic sculptures of India advocate that rudraksh of any facial variety can never do any harm to the wearer. Like the *Navrattanas* (nine planetary Gemstones), the rudraksh will have to be carefully chosen.

Another plus point in using rudraksh remedy is its life long permanent effect. A wearer can continue to use rudraksh irrespective of changes in the planetary positions. The continuous use of rudraksh can nullify the negative effects of malefic planets. Hence, various malefic effects identified in the horoscope can be cured by using specific facial variety of rudraksh. Onc of the most serious astrological problems called "Kal Sarp Yog" (KSY) can be effectively cured by using some specific combinations of rudraksh.

(5) Rudraksh as a perfect herbal medicine

Ancient medical science of India—the Ayurveda has extensively described the herbal healing miracles of rudraksh therapy for the holistic well-being of mankind.

Holy bead: Ayurveda recommends holy beads of rudraksh not only as contact therapy (by wearing etc) but also its multiple uses both as internal medicine in the form of powder (churan), incenerated ash (bhasm or vibhuti used both as external and internal medicine), oil, and emulsion, ointment extract in water or milk and also as an injection.

Leaves: The leaves of rudraksh tree are used for treating rheumatism and also serve as antidote to poison.

Fruit: The fruit of rudraksh is edible. The kernel or fleshy part of the fruit is sour in taste. It is eaten, pickled and even used in curries as a relishing food.

Apart from its food value, the fruit of rudraksh also has medicinal property.

(i) It is used as an effective medicine to cure fits of epilepsy.

(ii) It is also used in the treatment of gout, rheumatism, leprosy, dropsy, piles, ulcer and pneumonia.

(iii) It is emetic in its medicinal effect.

(6) Rudraksh Tree—A source of Quality Wood

The tree of rudraksh is a potential source of quality wood suitable for making—packing cakes, dugout, match boxes and splints.

The wood after finishing on it looks lustrous and shiny. It is also used for building, tea boxes and even for making charcoal.

(7) Rudraksh Pendulum used for analytical prediction and diagnosis of subtle energies

In the science of dowsing/radiesthesia (Satyavani vigyan)—the pendulum made from rudraksh bead gives quick and accurate diagnosis of diseases, disharmonies & also analytical divine predictions.

In the act of dowsing with rudraksh, a highly specialized subtle energy field is created which is called "cosmo-electromagnetic field". The swinging spectrum of this field emanates teletherapic messages which can be interpreted through the patterns of movement of the pendulum—called the language of dowsing.

(8) Rudraksh medication in psychosomatic diseases

The mental health problems like anxiety, anger, stress, illusion, delusion, possession syndrome due to evil effects etc. which are related to the waxing and waning of the moon cycle can be effectively cured by wearing a rudraksh mala of any facial variety, after its due purification and ritual activation.

During practice and research studies related to the effect of rudraksh on the excessive emotive behaviour/ hypersensitivity, I discovered the following specific observation:

"That wearing a long rosary of rudraksh which touches the level of naval region (i.e. just to save the waist level) is very effective cure for hyper sensitivity problems."

(9) Rudraksh remedy for removing Vastu defects

Since ages in India, a dwarbandhan made up of rudraksh is used to ward off the effects of negative vibrations. It removes all *Vastu doshas* in a residential or commercial building without any demolishing or renovation. Several experiential and experimental studies have verified the positive effects of dwarbandhans of rudraksh beads. It is also effective in curing 'Dristi dosh' and 'Ear dosh' which are inflicting negative vibrations. Such type of remedial vastu system which originated in ancient India is still widely practised in many houses of south India.

In making a dwarbhandhan, any facial variety can be selected. It should be made up of 54 beads of rudraksh and be tied inside the main door of the building.

Rudraksh beads are considered to be the source of purest form of cosmic energy which enhances positive vibrations. As an energetic herb, a genuine rudraksh is an inexhaustible source of pure cosmic energy. Inside your house or living room, drawing room or puja room, the photograph/statues of your revered deities should be adorned with a purified rosary of rudraksh. It enhances the spectrum of cosmic energy vibrations and positivity in your every living space & hence creates prosperity.

(10) Rudraksh as water purifier

The beads of rudraksh are best water purifier when kept for an hour in a pot containing potable water. As many as 2 to 5 rudrakshs can be kept in water as per capacity of the container. My experience has established that the best results of one rudraksh of any facial type are used for the purification of one litre of water. The rudraksh beads used once for water purification can be reused for next day. These beads can be used likewise for 40-days. However, after 40 days, it should not be used, because the potentials of the beads are exhausted after this period.

(11) Rudraksh water used as 'sacred bath' in spiritual healing.

The bath with rudraksh water is considered as sacred as a bath taken in the holy water of the Ganges. The bath should be taken by keeping nine rudraksh beads (preferably 3-faced) on head & pouring water on them—from head to downward onto the entire body.

(12) Rudraksh as panacea for holistic health, well-being and prosperity of life.

With enormous significance attached to the use of rudraksh, benefits for health, wealth, spiritual empowerment, mental peace, prosperity and success can be seen in all walks of life. Rudraksh beads are widely used as panacea for the cure of all ailments & evils in India & even abroad.

(13) Rudraksh for making sacred decorations and interior designs

The rudraksh beads made items used for decoration & interior designs are considered most auspicious and sacred.

Such products are also considered to be the integral sources of health, wealth, mental peace and well-being of mankind.

(14) Rudraksh therapy for deaddiction

The experiential studies have revealed that the rudraksh therapy is very helpful in shunning the bad habits of addiction due to alcohol and other narcotics. By wearing a rosary of genuine rudraksh, the spectrum of spiritual energy is enhanced so much so that the wearer attempts to get rid of addictions in due course of time.

Generally, it is advised to the wearer of a rudraksh rosary not to take wine, meat, garlic and onion. However, any therapeutic attempt to stick to vegetarianism and deaddiction would certainly reveal remarkable results.

●

Section III

RUDRAKSH THERAPY FOR PRACTICE, RESEARCH AND DEVELOPMENT

Chapter 5

Past And Present of Rudraksh Therapy: An Overview of Scientific Perspective

Milestones of Studies

The science of healing with herbal Rudraksh is as old as human civilization. In the nearly 5000 years old ancient Vedic scriptures of India and particularly Ayurveda, there are several references related to the healing potentials of Rudraksh.

Rudraksh healing as perfect therapy was widely practised in ancient India during Vedic period. As a safer, economical and easily available practice of Rudraksh therapy flourished not only in India and Nepal but also in several South Asian countries. Various religions all over the world realized the scientific validity of Rudraksh therapy for the cure and dynamization of the physical-mental-spiritual energies. Sages and the seers of all ages invariably used rudraksh for their spiritual empowerment and blissful consciousness. The review of available literature reveals that during the period of Vedic era and Mahabharata, the Rudraksh therapy was widely practised as system of traditional healing and complementary medicine for the holistic health, harmony and well-being of mankind.

The practice and research on ancient Rudraksh therapy could not grow enormously in India due to pre-independence period of slavery and disturbance for several years which was enjoyed by the foreign invaders and rulers. However, after independence in India the most recent contributions to the researches and publications were made in 1954 by Kirtikiran and Basu (1954) and Nandkarni (1954). Subsequently, more significant researches and publications were contributed by following researchers and authors:

Thayyril (1966); Dhar et al (1968); Sarkar et al (1972, 1973); Bhattacharya et al (1975); Chand (1975); Acharya (1976); Tripathi (1982); Gupta (1983); Pandey and Bhattacharya (1985); Raja (1987); David Lee (1991, 1997, 1998) and Shubhakaran (1997).

In 1966 Central Council of Ayurvedic Research, New Delhi published a book entitled "*Ayurvedic Oshadhi Nighantu*" by Kumaram Krishnan Thayyrial referring to several Rudraksh remedies. In the year 1968, a research team of Dr. M.L. Dhar and his associates carried out investigations on the screening of Indian medicinal plants including Rudraksh for biological activities. Further, in 1972 & 1973, noteworthy contributions on the medicinal potentials of Rudraksh were made by the research team of Dr. P.K. Sarkar and his associates.

In 1975, the research team of Dr. S.K. Bhattacharya carried out extensive research work into the pharmacological properties of Rudraksh. In the same year more interesting researches on the biochemical analysis of Rudraksh were published (Chand, 1975). Acharya (1976), contributed a book entitled *Shiv Puran* published by the Sanskrit Institute, Bareilly (UP) which carried several remarkable references on Rudraksh.

In 1982, both I.D. Tripathi and B. Tripathi contributed a book including significant references on Rudraksh remedies. In 1983, Dr. S.P. Gupta produced a masterly piece of research in the form of thesis for MD degree of Banares Hindu University, Varanasi (UP). More fillips to the scientific contributions on Rudraksh were further given by Dr. V.V. Pandey and Dr. S.K. Bhattacharya (1985), who published their noteworthy studies on "*Scientific Appraisal of Rudraksh*". This contribution revealed the analytical dimension of chemical and pharmacological potentials of Rudraksh. Raja (1987) described the medicinal properties of Rudraksh in the form of a comprehensive contribution on the subject.

Recently the more probing researches were carried out outside India by Dr. David Lee (1991, 97, 98) of the International University of Florida (USA). Dr. Lee worked out the detailed chemical analysis of Rudraksh and isolated some new active principles of high pharmacological efficacy. Even some pharmaceuticals in Belgium have also patented their injectable extracts derived from Rudraksh to effectively cure ailments related to heart and blood vascular system. Such investigations strongly endorse the more scientific validity of the holy bead of Rudraksh which have been remained as a popular healing system in India for more than 5 thousand years.

Efficacy of the Rudraksh Healing System

The mainstream system of western medicine so called allopathy has created a heavy influx of spurious drugs and their random use. This influx has caused tremendous stress on the natural human metabolism and has also much eroded the inbuilt human natural immunity (immune system). With the loss in the immunity, the health of human species has today not only been exposed to the ravages of scores of diseases of immune system but also staked its survival. If it goes unchecked the human species will be the first target of extinction in the hands of spurious drugs and unsafe unnatural medication. The only remedial recourse left with us to check the inflicting influx of spurious medicines is to make a rational use of allopathic medicines in combination with natural medicines and alternative therapies to gain & restore the holistic health of mankind.

Several alternative therapies / medicines have today been recommended by the World Health Organization (WHO). Yoga and many mind-body-healing systems including vibrative medicines have already been accepted by the World Health Organization (WHO) to cure and maintain the holistic level of health of mankind.

Rudraksh therapy widely practised, researched and developed in the Ayurvedic system of herbal medicine in India has been found effectively tested for the cure of ailments of heart, blood pressure and other blood vascular diseases, which are related to higher lever of cholesterol in the blood. Some other health problems for which Rudraksh therapy has been found effective are: *Allergy, psychosomatic & neurological diseases, asthma, diabetes and even some types of cancer*. It is essential to note that Rudraksh therapy should always been taken under the guidance of Rudraksh expert or Ayurvedic physician.

Scientific studies have revealed that the use of rudraksh in combination with other herbs brings quick and best results.

As a key system of treatment in Ayurveda, the Rudraksh remedies create a prefect balance of TRIDOSHA (vat, pit, and cough) & SEPTADOSHA which are essential components of the metabolism of human body.

Significance of Rudraksh Therapy

The highly specialized and significant features of Rudraksh Therapy are as under:

1. **Easy availability**: Due to abundant availability of the common varieties of Rudraksh, it can be made available to even a common man.
2. **Economic availability**: All the common varieties of Rudraksh are available at low cost on throw away price affordable by a common man.
3. **Higher longevity**: Due to higher longevity of the hardy holy bead of Rudraksh, its potential can be used for a longer time. Hence, it is a permanent and life long panacea for all ills and evils.
4. **Safer use:** The use of Rudraksh is always safer without any side effects / contraindications.
5. **Easily practicable**: The system of healing through Rudraksh is easily practicable even by a layman for self and trans-healing.
6. **Preventive and curative action**: In the cure of all illnesses, the mode of therapeutic action of Rudraksh is both preventive and curative.

How Rudraksh Cures?

Process of Healing

The remedial usage of Rudraksh therapy not only cures illness but also promotes health and longevity. It protects and restores natural immunity of the body. The mode of therapeutic healing of Rudraksh involves its special *physical, chemical and electromagnetic attributes.*

1. ***Healing based on physical features (Morphological attributes)***

1. *Herbal acupressure effect on neurophysiology:* The surface of rudraksh has roughage due to several natural uneven projections on it. These acu-points influence a natural acupressure effect on the nerve endings (neurophysiology) and stimulate them to release their secretions which restore the health and harmony.

2. *Herbal thermoregulation effect:* The entire surface of rudraksh bears several thousand micropores (thermopiles). Both experimental and experiential studies have found that these micropores suck the excessive heal of the body and release it to the outside, hence a rudraksh performs a thermoregulatory functions. This attribute saves the health from the inflictions due to higher rise of body temperature. This also cures the problem of hypertension high blood pressure. Excessive rise in blood pressure is induced due to thermo effects which are prevented and cured.

3. *Healing based on chemical composition.* (Chemo-elemental attributes): Researches have confirmed that due to its specific chemo-pharmacological properties, the rudraksh can be widely used as: Cardiac stimulant, anti-cholesterol, depressant of CNS, relaxant of smooth muscles, immunity enhancer, energizer of our bio-energy field (aura) and meridian centers (energetic chakra system).

The biological properties include its special effects as anti-viral, anti-bacterial, anti-cancerous, anti-fungal, anti-protozoal & anti-helminthic.

4. *Healing based on electromagnetic properties (Electromagnetic attributes)*

Researches have established that the herbal beads of Rudraksh have dia-electric attributes because they store the impulses of electrical energy and have permanent magnetic properties. They are electromagnetic, paramagnetic in nature. Rudraksh beads are also known to have dynamic polarity or the ability to change polarity.

The pendulum like swinging action of the pendant of rudraksh shunts excessive negative energies (Ohm's Law) which are harmful to our metabolism and restores required positive energy from the cosmos.

Hence, Rudraksh restores a perfect balance of electromagnetic impulses which are optimally required for the health and harmony of our life.

●

Chapter 6

Rudraksh Remedies in Astrology for Health Care

Rudraksh in astrology as Zodiacal Therapy

Astrology is the ancient divine science related to the language of cosmic energy and its effects on all life forms. In more explicit term, it should be understood that Astrology is basically all about the patterns of cosmic and biocosmic energy vibrations, the interpretation of their vital effects, their manifestation and management to harness the maximum benefits for the peace and prosperity of mankind.

In several advanced countries including Russia where Astrology was explored more scientifically, it is called BIOCOSMIC SCIENCE or COSMOBIOLOGY.

In Astrology and Ayurveda, the ancient science of life, originated in India is the oldest system of medicinc. Several references have been made on the Astro-medical benefits of rudraksh therapy. A review of available ancient scriptures of India reveals that the rudraksh therapy was widely practised in India as a most popular traditional healing system. The remedial applications of rudraksh in the light of modern researches expand the horizons of effective use of rudraksh in physical therapies or contact therapies and promote its importance in complementary medicines.

Astral-Remedies based on facial varieties of Rudraksh

The facial varieties of Rudraksh are based on the number of vertical furrows or longitudinal grooves on the surface of it. The grooves are also called faces or mukhs of rudraksh.

In astrology, the remedial use of rudraksh is based on its facial types (varieties). Some specific human ailments are treated by specific facial varieties.

In the ancient Indian Vedic and puranic scriptures as many as 38 facial varieties of rudraksh have been described. The faceless rudraksh (Nirankars) which is devoid of longitudinal furrows are rarely available and are much powerful in their effectiveness.

However, nowadays the available species of rudraksh are referable to only 1-14 facial varieties. Studies have revealed that the Rudraksh of 15-21 faces (mukhis) are very rare and hence costly and most of the rudraksh of 28-31 faces (mukhis) are not available.

Description of various faces of Rudraksh, their relationship with Astrological Zodiac signs, Diseases and their cure for life prosperity

1. ***One faced Rudraksh (Eka Mukhi):***
   (Single longitudinal furrow);
   Ruling planet: Sun (Apollo):

Diseases cured: Ailments of eyes, heart, blood circulation, blood-pressure, nervous system, bones, vitamin A&D deficiency, night blindness, stomatitis & appendicitis.

Additional benefits: It removes negativity of thoughts and enhances total prosperity. It also gives total fulfilment of all aspirations of life and blesses with spiritual bliss and empowerment.

Spiritual significance: As per Hindu belief, this rudraksh variety is incarnation of Lord Shiva and very rarely available. Hence, it is also called *Shiva Rudraksh.* For getting equal benefits, its alternate is 11 faced rudraksh (Eka Dasha Mukhi).

How to use: As a rosary or wearing a single Rudraksh on any Monday gives most effective benefits. It should be used after due ritual purification and activation.

2. ***Two Faced Rudraksh (Dwi-Mukhi):***
   (Two longitudinal furrows)
   Ruling planet: - Moon

Diseases cured: Best cure for the ailments of lungs, kidneys, digestive system, heart and blood circulation, memory, fatness & obesity. It cures menstrual disorders & infertility and also useful in chronic cough and rhinitis.

Additional benefits: (1) The use of two faced rudraksh is a powerful remedy against the malefic effects of deflected moon which causes high blood pressure.

(2) The wearing of rudraksh (single or rosary) helps the wearer to have a control of desires. It also enhances the spectrum of spiritual energy and awakening of Kundalini power.

(3) It blesses the wearer a dynamic bio-magnetic aura field (vashikaran) to dominate over others.

(4) It is an effective cure for the loss or depletion of memory.

Spiritual significance: It is *Ardha Nareeshwara* incarnation referable to Lord Shiva and Parvati together.

How to use: Wearing a single rudraksh studded in silver or a rosary bearing 51 or 108 beads is potentially effective. It should be worn on any Monday after ritual purification and activation. A rosary or single rudraksh in black or white thread is effective cure for high blood pressure.

3. *Three Faced Rudraksh (Tri-Mukhi):*
(Three longitudinal furrows):
Ruling Planet: Mars:

Diseases cured : Indigestion, piles, ulcers, diseases of eyes, asthma, testes enlargement, heart diseases and high blood pressure. It also cures anemia, malaria and other health problems related to abortion, menstruation, emotional imbalances and mental anxiety.

Additional benefits: It helps in the achievement of higher education, career opportunities etc.

Spiritual significance: This variety of rudraksh is regarded as incarnation of God of Agni or Fire. It also blesses the benedictions of Brahma, Vishnu & Mahesh as per Indian religious philosophy.

How to use: It should be used as a single bead or a rosary in red or pink thread for getting maximum benefits of its potentials.

4. *Four Faced Rudraksh (Chatur Mukhi)*
(Four longitudianal furrows):
Ruling Planet: Mercury

Diseases cured: Asthma, jaundice, sinusitis, epilepsy skin diseases, mental and memory problems.

Additional benefits: Best for increasing mind and memory potentials.

Spiritual significance:: (1) Wear a rosary or a single bead of four faced rudraksh with red thread like the necklace.

(2) A single four faced rudraksh worn in green thread on any wednesday is effective in the cure of asthma.
(3) For internal use, this rudraksh should be boiled with milk (one glass)...cool, and take it for 21 days regularly. This remedy is effective in the cure of above cited diseases.

5. *Five Faced Rudraksh (Panch Mukhi): (Fig. 2)*
(Five longitudinal furrows):
Ruling planet: Jupiter

Diseases cured: Disorders of liver, bone, fat, kidney and arthritis. It also cures sexual diseases and diabetes. It is preventive to heart diseases and normalizes the high blood-pressure fluctuations.

Additional benefits: Best for settlement of instability in health, wealth and spiritual life. It is also protective against evil effects and enhances mental peace and life prosperity.

Spiritual significance: It is *kalagni swaroop* and Rudranga hence has much spiritual significance.

How to use:: (1) Wearing a rosary or a single bead in yellow thread is effective in action.
(2) To wear a single five mukhi rudraksh in red or pink thread on any sunday is most effective in the cure of all heart ailments in particular.
(3) Keeping a five mukhi rudraksh in a copper glass containing water and keep it soaked for the over-night. Take this rudraksh soaked water every day in the morning and repeat it for 21 days. It cures all chronic heart diseases and also detoxes (purifies) the blood.

6. *Six faced rudraksh (Shan mukhi):*
(Six longitudianal furrows)
Ruling Planet: Venus

Diseases cured: All diseases of reproductive system, sexual disorders, urinary system, stomatitis, ailments of throat and eye. It is best for chest pains and women diseases (hysteria, fits and epilepsy etc.).

Additional benefits: (1) It enhances awareness for dominance and harmonization of body, mind, and soul energies, hence gives holistic consciousness.
(2) It expands and sharpens the potentials of the mind and memory. Hence, it is best for students in particular.

Spiritual significance: It is incarnation of Lord Kartikeya.

How to use: Wearing a rosary or a single bead of six faced rudraksh in white thread will give effective results. It enhances the confidence power of eloquence (effective speech).

7. *Seven Faced Rudraksh (Saptha Mukhi):*
(Seven longitudinal furrows)
Ruling Planet: Saturn

Diseases cured: Cataract of eyes, skin and sexual disorders including impotency, delirium, fickle mindedness (lack of confidence) and diseases of respiratory system.

Additional benefits: (1) It enhances wealth resources hence, best for the growth of money.

(2) It wards-off risks of accident and enmity.

(3) It is known to have high power of hypnosis which it blesses to its wearers.

Spiritual significance: It is incarnation of Lord Manmadha also called Ananga.

How to use: A rosary of single bead of seven faced rudraksh in blue or black thread is most effective in results. The much preferred use of it is to keep in cash box for the prosperity of wealth resources.

8. *Eight Faced Rudraksh (Astha Mukhi):*
(Eight longitudinal furrows)
Ruling planet: Rahu

Diseases cured : Diseases of eyes, testes, skin, lungs, liver and spleen. It is also effective in the early stages of paralysis.
(2) It is especially effective in the cure of enlargement of liver and spleen for which it should be used with red thread around the neck or tie on your right arm.

Additional benefits : (1) Best for enhancing intelligence, memory, mind power (concentration & confidence).

(2) It is effective in setting the problems of career and also success in litigation.

Spiritual significance : It is incarnation of Lord Ganesh.

How to use : It should be used as a single bead or a rosary. Only red thread should be used along with it.

9. *Nine Faced Rudraksh (Nava Mukhi): (Fig. 3)*
(Nine longitudinal furrows)
Ruling planet : Ketu

Diseases cured : Diseases of heart, lungs, eyes, stomach, skin, small-pox, miscarriages and abortions, childlessness.

Additional benefits: It wards-off risks of accident, enmity and evil effects.

Spiritual significance : It is incarnation of Lord Bhairava/ main deity of Goddess Durga.

How to use : Wearing a rosary or a single bead in grey or black thread is effective in action.

10. *Ten faced Rudraksh (Dasha Mukhi):*
(Ten longitudinal furrows)
Ruling planet : Jupiter

Diseases cured : It is panacea for all health problems. It also stabilizes the total health of mind, body, soul energies. In particular, it is special remedy for whooping cough, anxiety and mental tension.

Additional benefits : It is best for settlement of career and also signifies the spiritual power.

Spiritual significance : It is incarnation of Lord Vishnu and also called Janardhana.

How to use : Wearing a rosary or single bead of ten faced rudraksh in black or yellow thread gives effective results.

11. *Eleven faced Rudraksh (Ekadasha Mukhi):*
(Eleven longitudinal furrows)
Ruling planet :- Sun

Diseases cured : It cures all women diseases and in particular infertility/childlessness.

Additional benefits : It is preventive as well as curative in its effectivity with regard to all diseases of women.

Spiritual significance : It is incarnation of Lord Rudra (Shiva) and is best alternative for the one faced rudraksh which is rarely available.

How to use : A single bead or a rosary of this rudraksh in combination with red thread is best in its effectivity. Experiential studies have revealed that much satisfactory results can be obtained if this rudraksh is worn on forehead.

12. *Twelve faced Rudraksh : (Dwadasha Mukhi):*
(Twelve longitudinal furrows)
Ruling planet : Adi Devta (Sun)

Diseases cured : It is very effective for chronic diseases and prolonged ailments in particular Jaundice.

Additional benefits : It improves confidence, memory and mental powers. It is best for the control of excessive sexual desire and also perverted habits and fickle mindedness.

Spiritual significance : It is incarnation of Maha Vishnu and Adi Devta (Sun), hence it is also called Aditya.

How to use : It should be worn as a single bead or a rosary in combination with red thread.

13. *Thirteen faced Rudraksh : (Trayodasha Mukhi): (Thirteen longitudinal furrows) Ruling planet : Venus*

Diseases cured : It cures all the ailments of urinary system and also the reproductive system. It is best for the treatment of skin and sexual disorders. It is more effective in the cure of some early stages of cancer and also the diseases of eyes, ears, nose and throat (E.E.N.T.) Experiential studies has revealed that the proper use of this rudraksh is best for ladies who fulfill their aspirations of health, feature, figure and beauty.

Additional benefits : It enhances mind and memory powers and also the sense of creativity, hence much useful for the students and career oriented persons.

Spiritual significance : It is incarnation of Lord Indra.

How to use :- It can be used both as a single bead or rosary in combination with white, blue thread.

14. *Fourteen faced Rudraksh : (Chaturdasha Mukhi): (Fourteen longitudinal furrows): (Fig. 4) Ruling planet : Saturn*

Diseases cured : It is best for the cure of partial facial paralysis. It is also effective for the cure of anxiety and depression.

Additional benefits : It restores general health and wellness. It blesses peace, prosperity and wealth aspirations.

Spiritual significance : It is incarnation of Lord Param Shiva and prathika of Lord Hanuman.

How to use : It should bc used as a single bead or rosary in combination with black or red thread. Much better results can be obtained, if it is worn on forehead.

Holistic Healing with Rudraksh Rosary

How to make a rosary of Rudraksh?

It is generally made with red or black silk thread and sometime with white cotton thread also. Preferably, the colour of thread should be as per the zodiacal sign of the ruling planet. For getting more benefits of effectivity the wires of gold, silver and even copper are also used in accordance to its specifically prescribed use. When made in copper, it should be kept clean regularly to avoid the formation of greenish blue colour of copper oxide.

Number of holy beads

The number of holy beads of rudraksh in a rosary is variable as per its placement on any part of the body as contact therapy. The prescribed auspicious number of rudraksh beads in a rosary is given in the following table. It is essential to avoid the use of rudraksh for making rosary if it is defaced, much thorny and eaten by worms/insects and has broken faces (longitudinal lines on the surface).

Table : 1

Number of beads of rudraksh rosary and their spiritual significance for life prosperity is as under

Number	Significant effects
100	Blesses with Salvation
140	Blesses with freedom from desires.
108	Blesses with success in all walks of life.
32	Blesses with wealth & fulfillment of aspirations for financial resources.

Table : 2

The number of Rudraksh beads to be used on various parts of the body for effective benefits

Body Organs/Parts	Number of beads	Sources
Shikha (Crown hair)	1	Srimaddevibhagavata
Wrist (both)	12/12	– do –
Neck	31	– do –
Forehead	40	– do –
Ears (both)	6/6	– do –
Chest	108	– do –
Shoulders	500	– do –
Yajnopaveet (sacred thread)	108	– do –
Neck	2 rows	– do –
Other parts of the body, Viz. ear ring (*kundal*) Crown, ear ornament, Kangan waist (*Mekhala*), Abdomen etc.	3 rows	– do –
Crown	550	Siva Purana
Crown	1100	– do –
Yajnopaveet (sacred thread)	360 (3 rows)	– do –
Sikha (crown hair)	1 & 3	– do –
Ears (both)	6/6	– do –

Neck	101, 50, 32,	– do –
Fore-arm (both)	11, 16, 24	– do –
Karpoor dvara	11	– do –
Wrists (both)	11; 12	– do –
Yajnopaveet (sacred thread)	3 strings each of 108	– do –
Waist region	5	– do –
Forehead	30, 40	– do –
Shoulders	500	– do –
Heart (chest)	108	– do –
Sikha (Crown hair)	1	Rudraksajabalo-panisad
Forehead	30	– do –
Neck region	36	– do –
Fore arms (both)	16/16	– do –
Wrist (both)	12/12	– do –
Shoulders	15	– do
Yajnopaveet (sacred thread)	108	– do –
Neck region	2, 3, 5 & 7 rows	– do –
Crown	-	– do –
Kundal (ear ring)	-	– do –
Ear ornament	-	– do –
Wrists	-	– do –
Waist	-	– do –
	300 (mean)	– do –
	500 (medium)	– do –
	1000 (best)	
Eyes (both)	4/4	Padarthaparsa nirnayasindhu
Neck region	32	– do –
Forehead	40	– do –
Ear (both)	6/6	– do –
Wrists (both)	12/12	– do –
Fore arms (both)	16/16	– do –
Sikha (crown hair)	1	– do –
Heart (chest)	108	– do –

Various Astrological prescriptions are given in Table 3 - 6.

Table : 3

Astrological Prescriptions of Rudraksh as per Birth-Lagna and Birth Rashi

Birth Rashi/Lagna	Ruling Planet	Prescribed Rudraksh For the Rashi
1. Mesha (Aries)	Mercury	Three Mukhi
2. Vrisabha (Taurus)	Venus	Six Mukhi
3. Mithun (Gemini)	Mercury	Four Mukhi
4. Karka (Cancer)	Moon	Two Mukhi
5. Singh (Leo)	Sun	One or Twelve Mukhi
6. Kanya (Virgo)	Mercury	Four Mukhi
7. Tula (Libra)	Venus	Six Mukhi
8. Vrishchika (Scorpio)	Mars	Three Mukhi
9. Dhanu (Sagittarius)	Jupiter	Five Mukhi
10. Makar (Capricorn)	Saturn	Seven Mukhi
11. Kumbha (Aquarius)	Saturn	Seven Mukhi
12. Meena (Pisces)	Jupiter	Five Mukhi

Table : 4

Astrological Prescriptions of Rudraksh as per Nakshatra in Horoscope

S. No.	Birth Nakshatra	Ruling Planet	Rudraksh Prescribed
1.	Ashwani	Ketu	Nine Mukhi
2.	Bharani	Venus	Six Mukhi
3.	Kritika	Sun	One, Twelve or Eleven Mukhi
4.	Rohini	Moon	Two Mukhi
5.	Mrigashira	Mars	Three Mukhi
6.	Ardra	Rahu	Eight Mukhi
7.	Punarvasu	Jupiter	Five Mukhi
8.	Pushya	Saturn	Seven Mukhi
9.	Ashlesha	Mercury	Four Mukhi
10.	Magha	Ketu	Nine Mukhi
11.	Purvaphalguni	Venus	Six Mukhi
12.	Uttaraphalguni	Sun	One, Twelve, Eleven Mukhi
13.	Hasta	Moon	Two Mukhi

14. Chitra	Mars	Three Mukhi
15. Swati	Rahu	Eight Mukhi
16. Vishakha	Jupiter	Five Mukhi
17. Anuradha	Saturn	Seven Mukhi
18. Jeystha	Mercury	Four Mukhi
19. Mula	Ketu	Nine Mukhi
20. Purvshadha	Venus	Six Mukhi
21. Uttarashadha	Sun	One, Twelve, Eleven Mukhi
22. Shravana	Moon	Two Mukhi
23. Dhanishta	Mars	Three Mukhi
24. Shatabhistha	Rahu	Eight Mukhi
25. Purvabhadrapada	Jupiter	Seven Mukhi
26. Uttarabhadrapada	Saturn	Seven Mukhi
27. Revati	Mercury	Four Mukhi

Table : 5

Colour varieties of Rudraksh which can best be recommended for various zodiac signs in Astrology

Colour of Rudraksh	Useful in Zodiacal Science (Rashi)	Ruling Planet
White or Brown	1. Cancer (Kark)	Moon (Chandrama)
	2. Pisces (Meen)	Jupiter (Brihaspati)
	3. Taurus (Brish)	Venus (Shukra)
Yellow	1. Aries (Mesh)	Mars (Mangal)
	2. Leo (Singh)	Sun (Surya)
	3. Sagittarius (Dhanu)	Jupiter (Brahaspati)
Red	1. Scorpio (Brischek)	Mars (Mangal)
	2. Virgo (Kanya)	Mercury (Budh)
	3. Capricorn (Makar)	Saturn (Shani)
Black	1. Gemini (Mithun)	Mercury (Budh)
	2. Libra (Tula)	Venus (Shukra)
	3. Aquarius (Kumbh)	Saturn (Shani)

Table : 6

Guidelines for the beneficial use of Rudrakash as per birth date and phonetically beneficial alphabets

Birth date range	Zodical sign		Zodic Planet	Phonetics of Beneficial alphabets	Rudrakash to be used as per No. of faces	
	Rashi (Hindi)	Zodic (English)			Specific face	Alternate faces
20 March-19 April	Mekh	Aries	Mars (Mangal)	Chu, che, cho, la, li, lu, lu, le, lo, aa	3	1, 9
20 April-20 May	Brikh	Taurus	Venus (Shukra)	u, ee, e, wa, wi, wv, wo	5	2, 4, 6, 10
21 May-22 June	Mithun	Gemini	Mercury (Budh)	ka, ki, ku, gha, Angha chha, ke, ko, ha	4	3, 11, 14
23 June-21 July	Karak	Cancer	Moon (Chandrama)	hi, ha, hu, ho, da, di, dhu, de, doo	2	4, 7, 12
22 July-22August	Singh	Leo	Sun (Surya)	ma, mi, mu, me, mo, ta ts, tii, too, tee	1	5, 9, 12, 14
23 Aug.-21 Sept.	Kanya	Virgo	Mercury (Budh)	to, pi, pu, sha, ara, tha, pe, po	4	6, 10, 13
22 Sept.-22 Oct.	Tula	Libra	Venus (shukra)	ra, ri, ru, re, ro, ta, ti, tu, te	6	3, 7, 11, 13
23 oct.-21 nov.	Brischik	Scorpio	Mars (Mangal)	to, na, ni, nu, ne, no, ya, yi, yu	3	4, 6, 8, 12
22 Nov.-22 Dec.	Dhanu	Sagittarius	Jupiter (Brihaspati)	ye, yo, bha, bhi, bhu, dha, pha, hha, sha	5	1, 9
23 Dec.-20 Jan.	Makar	Capricorn	Saturn (Shani)	bho, jha, ji, ju, jo, je, kha, khi, khoo, ga; gi	7	5, 8, 10, 13
21 Jan.-19 Feb.	Kumbh	Aquarius	Saturn (Shani)	gu, gi, go, sa, si, su, sa, so, da	7	2, 11
20 Feb.-19March	Meen	Pisces	Jupiter (Brihaspati)	di, du, tha, jha, yina, de, do, choo, cha	5	8, 12, 14

Cleansing and purification of rudraksh rosary

Cleansing: It is essential to clean the Rudraksh rosary every month. It should be cleaned with simple water or Gangajal (Ganges water). Due to body sweat and dirt particles the natural pores of rudraksh are clogged which can be cleaned by using any clean tooth brush and water. This process keeps upon the micropores in rudraksh which are essential for the passage of healing energy. The author has observed that the best way to keep rudraksh clean is to keep it in soap-nut water (Reetha water) for two hours and clean it with a tooth-brush. After using a rudraksh as medicine in lukewarm or hot warm milk it should be properly washed and cleaned in soap-nut water. By not doing so, the milk soaked in rudraksh attracts flies, fungus, bacteria, etc. which spoil its further use, hence the cleaning is most essential.

Purification: Rudraksh can be purified and worn again by washing it with pure sandal wood paste, coconut water, milk, curd, ghee, honey and finally it should be washed with clean water (preferably under fast running tap water).

The purification can be done once in a month. However, the application of sandal-wood, sindoor and vibhuti smeard on rudraksh and not washed away frequently reduces its longevity and also effectivity. At least once in a month a periodic cleaning and purification of rosary of the rudraksh must be done. The experiential study of the author has shown that the washing of rudraksh in liquid soap under running tap water is more effective. After washing, it should be dried with any soft cloth made up of muslin or cotton. The rudraksh dried properly should be smeared with sandal wood paste/mustard oil which enhances its preservation, glow and effectivity.

Who should wear rudraksh?: The holy bead of rudraksh can be worn by the people of all castes, creeds and religions invariably. There is no gender discrimination for wearing rudraksh. Both males and females can wear the rosary and can get equally effective benefits. However, it should not be worn by the ladies during menstrual period and by both male and female during sexual act.

When to wear rudraksh?: After due cleaning and purification, the rudraksh should be worn on any Monday,

Amavasya (half moon day), Purnima (full moon day) or Mahashivratri (International Rudraksh Day).

How to wear rudraksh?: Before wearing rudraksh, the worship of Lord Shiva should be done as per ritual. The rudraksh should be touched to the SHIVLINGA and chanting of the mantra 'OM NAMAH SHIVAYA' should be exercised for 108 times. The rosary of rudraksh spiritualized as such works very effectively as an energized remedy to fulfill all aspirations of the wearer.

In order to get the health benefits and get rid of diseases the rosary of rudraksh (Fig. 7 & 8) should be energized and spiritualized by chanting 108 times the vibrations of MAHA MRITTHUNJAY MANTRA cited below.

Sanskrit version

In English: *"Om thryambakam yajamache sugonthim pushti vardham urvasuka meva bandana, Mruthyor Mrikshiya Maamruthath"*

Process of Jaap prayers with rudraksh rosary

A rosary of rudraksh to be used for jaap prayers should not be used for wearing and healing the ailments. A rosary for jaap should therefore, always be a separate one. The smallest jaap mala (rosary) should have 27 beads and not less than it. Every rosary should not be shared with other person for the jaap.

In every rosary of rudraksh, there is a single additional rudraksh called *Meru* or *Sand Yothambija*. This point is an indicator of the end of 108 beads of rudraksh in a single rosary. It is always outside the circuits of 108 beads.

During prayers, the NERU point should not be crossed in the continuity of beads. For recounting once again on reaching the NERU point the counting should be reversed. If the number of holy beads of rudraksh in a rosary is 54 it should be counted twice to get the desired target of 108 jaaps.

Time and process for rudraksh Jaap

The jaap prayers with rudraksh can be performed three times a day for which the process is as under:-

Morning Jaap: It should be completed before 10 A.M. During this jaap, mala (rosary) should be at the level of nabhi (umbilicus/navel region).

Benefits: It prevents and cures all diseases of stomach and abdomen.

Afternoon Jaap : It should be performed between 10 A.M. (noon) and 2.30 P.M. (afternoon). During this jaap, the rosary should be held at the level of chest and heart.

Benefits: It prevents and cures all diseases of chest and heart.

Evening Jaap: It should be performed between 4 P.M. to 7 P.M. During this jaap, rosary should be kept at the level of rose point.

Benefits: It prevents and cures the diseases of respiratory system, like asthma, bronchitis and pneumonia etc.

Benefits of Rudraksh Rosary

A pure & purified pre-energized rudraksh rosary of 108 holy beads is most powerful and beneficial. Its benefits are described as under:

(1) It fulfills all aspirations of the wearer related to health, wealth, peace, prosperity, name and fame.

(2) As a powerful remedy, it is a panacea for all ailments in general & in particular for the diseases of heart, blood vascular system & the nervous system. It is especially effective for the quick & permanent cure of high blood pressure/hypertension.

(3) According to Tantric school of thoughts, the wearing of rosary of rudraksh blesses the wearer with special spiritual & supernatural powers of Ridhis & Sidhis. Such like powers are also known to be found in the rosary of beads of tulsi plant (ocinum sanctum) which is known to its wearer with special psychic power called Sidhi.

(4) Rudraksh rosary is most effective in getting maximum benefits from the jaap & also vandyavandanam etc.

(5) Wearing a rudraksh rosary or even a single rudraksh after due purification always keeps off evil effects & also the afflictions due to the malefic planets. Hence, the rudraksh is a perfect system of healing all the "ills & evils".

(6) Experiential & experimental studies have revealed that the rosary of rudraksh is known to enhance the spectrum of creative subtle images (positivity) & spiritual empowerment.

Wearing a rosary of 108 holy beads helps in the fast activation & dynamization of the kundalini energy (serpent power) during meditation.

It not only enhances the quantum level and subtle energy of the body but also quickens the state of blissfulness during meditation.

●

Chapter 7

Rudraksh Therapy in Ayurveda for Healthcare and Life Prosperity

Rudraksh as a therapy cures a disease not only at physical, mental and emotional level but also strengthens the vital life force (bioenergetic system) enhancing natural vigour, self-confidence, intelligence, intuition and memory system. It creates a holistic balance in the natural health and harmony of life.

Medicinal Potentials of Rudraksh

Chemical composition of rudraksh: An overview of researches

In the recent year, the significance of medicinal potentials of rudraksh has been much enhanced due to researches which yielded astounding results related to the chemical composition and pharmacological uses of the active principles in rudraksh.

In the new era, one of the earliest known references on Rudraksh studies was done by John Garret (1864). Subsequently, a complete botanical survey of Rudraksh was undertaken by Lt. Col. Kerber Drory. Researches on rudraksh were further expanded by the studies of Mr. Paul Hume – an Englishman, who concluded that:

"Nothing is impossible for a Rudraksh remedy because it can change the wearer's health condition, fate and hypnotizes people based upon its method of usage."

Col. R.N. Chopra who lived his life as one of the foremost researches and contributions on Indian Medicinal Plants also described the medicinal potentials of Rudraksh. In his extensive contribution on the *Glossary of Indian medicinal plants* he refers at *p. 105* that "*Rudraksh fruits are used in the treatment of Neurological diseases. On the basis of pharmacological experiments, it was claimed that Rudraksh works on Central Nervous System (CNS) and acts as : depressant, relaxant of smooth muscles, hypertensive, hypoglycemic and cardiac stimulant.*"

Both in India and abroad, several research investigations on the chemical analysis and pharmacological properties have greatly enhanced the scientific validity of Rudraksh therapy as a traditional and complementary medicine system.

Most comprehensive research on Rudraksh at Central Institute of Ayurveda, Kolkata were carried out by Dhar et al (1968). Analysis of chemical composition revealed some remarkable active principles and their usage for the treatment of head *diseases, epileptic fits and asthma.* Some active principles isolated from Rudraksh during researches are:

1. Palmatic acid
2. Isopalmatic acid
3. Linoleic acid
4. Myristic acid.

The research team also identified some pigments, *oil droplets* and *crystals of calcium oxalate* as constituents of Rudraksh.

Some reports related to the Physio-chemical composition of Rudraksh are as under (Table 7 & 8) :-

Table : 7

Physio-chemical composition of Rudraksh

Water moisture	:	8.87%
Oil contents	:	0.68%
Colour of oil	:	pale yellow
Consistency	:	liquid
Refractive index	:	1.4650
Specific gravity	:	0.9300
Sponification value	:	176.30
Sponification equivalent	:	317.80
IV	:	73.28
AV	:	34.89
Unsponified matter	:	03.76

Table : 8

Chemical analysis of Rudraksh water

Periodic duration	Sample-I	Sample-II
After 24 hours		
(1) PH	4.82	
(2) Chemical oxygen Demand (COD)	4,800 mg/lit	200mg/lit
(3) Electrical Conductivity (EC)	PH 5.8 EC = 1535	375 (EC)
After 48 hours		
(1) pH 4.8	—	pH 5.7
(2) COD	152mg/lit	11.2mg/lit
(3) EC	665	60

Further contributions on the chemical composition of rudraksh were made by Sarkar et al (1972, 1973), Bhattacharya et al (1973), Chand (1975), Gupta (1983), Pandey and Bhattacharya (1985) and published excellent studies related to the scientific appraisal revealing its chemical and pharmacological potentials. Researches on the chemical composition of rudraksh have now been extended beyond India. Dr. David Lee of the International University of Florida extensively worked out the active principles of rudraksh and their pharmacological efficacy (1998).

Table : 9

Chemical analysis of the edible part of the drupe of Rudraksh (from Ceylon) investigated the following values (Flora British India Vol. I p.401).

Analysis of drupe of Rudraksh (*Elaeocarpus serratus*)

Moisture	:	77.2%
Crude protein	:	0.69%
Total carbohydrates	:	19.53%
Total sugar	:	9.8%
Ether extract	:	0.46%
Fibre	:	1.49%
Mineral matter	:	0.59%
Vitimin-C	:	47 mg/100g. (mainly due to citric acid).

Table : 10

Chemical analysis of seeds of Rudraksh revealed fixed oil contents with following constants: (Flora British India Vol. I p.401).

$d_4 15^o$	:	0.9067
$n_D 15^o$	:	1.4671
Sap val	:	192.52
Iod val	:	82.66
Acid val	:	3.56

Table : 11

Microanalysis of Rudraksh bead based on chemical composition and water test for ten hours in the laboratory of Chemical Technology Department, University of Mumbai (Bhatia, 2001).

Content		**Percentage**
Carbon	:	45.3%
Hydrogen	:	5.8%
Nitrogen	:	1.0%
Water Test		
pH	:	5.8
sulphur	:	00
Hydrogen	:	0.0

Laboratory tests also reveal the presence of Vitamin-C which is essential for the maximization of immunity of the body.

Table : 12

Nutritional value of Rudraksh Fruit (David W. Lee 1998)

Carbohydrates	:	21.0% (Dry mass) or 0.58 g. per fruit
Proteins	:	4.3% (Dry mass) or 0.12 g. per fruit

Table : 13

Fatty Acid composition in Rudraksh.

Constituent	**Composition**
ISO Palmiatic fatty acud	8.0
ISO stearic fatty acid	18.1 – 18.2
Oil	0.2
Steam Distilled Products	14.18
Traces	NIL.

Some other physical Parameters are given in Table 14

Table : 14

Some Physical Parameters of Rudraksh (Subas Rai, 2004)

Mukhi	Specific Gravity	PH of Extract	wt. gm.
1.	1.2	4.48	5.34
2.	1.2	5.76	4.77
3.	1.5	7.96	1.85
4.	1.3	7.4	3.19
5. (small)	1.8	7.52	0.64
(large)	-	6.78	2.57
6.	1.09	6.45	3.60
7.	1.5	5.97	3.51
8.	1.08	6.74	3.63
9.	1.05	6.58	6.37
10.	1.2	6.87	6.87
11.	1.2	6.57	7.03
12.	1.4	6.50	4.26
13.	1.5	6.55	- 7.65
14.	1.6	4.9	- 7.25

Pharmacological & Biological properties of Rudraksh

Pharmacological properties

Bio-pharmacological researches on rudraksh revealed several medicinal properties. Based on the effect of active principles on the human physiology and metabolism, the following medicinal properties have been identified in rudraksh–

1. **Cardiac stimulant** : It protects heart from depression and hence serves as a cardiac booster.
2. **Anti-cholcstcrol** : It checks the higher level of fats (lipids) in the blood. Besides, it protects us from cardio-vascular diseases like heart attack, strokes, angina, arteriosclerosis and myocardial infraction.
3. **Depressant of CNS:** (Central Nervous System) : It suppresses the over-excited phase of nerves and hence releases the stress. As an effective stress buster it cures various *neurological diseases*.
4. **Relaxant of smooth muscles & energizer of our Aura (Bio-energy field) and Bio-energy centers including Meridians (Chakra system):**
   As a relaxant of smooth muscles, it releases the mental stress psychosomatically. Hence, it creates relaxed state of mind and attitude. It energizes our bio-energy field.

5. **Immunity Enhancer :** As a source of vitamin-C, it maximizes the immunity of the body. The activation and dynamization of our immune system give us an effective defense against all dreadful diseases like AIDS, cancer etc. Hence, rudraksh is an effective, preventive & curative remedy.
6. **Hypotensive :** This property regulates and monitors the high blood pressure. Rudraksh remedy is highly prophylactic against hypertensive syndrome.
7. **Hypoglycemic :** This property regulates and monitors the higher level of sugar in the blood. Hence, due to this efficacy the rudraksh remedy is effective against diabetes.
8. **Anti-convulsant** : Due to this property, rudraksh is effective in the cure of diseases like epilepsy and other neurological disorders.
9. **Anti-pyretic** : This property controls high fever and maintains the normal natural temperature of the body. Due to such an efficacy the rudraksh is effective as a thermo-regulatory remedy.

Biological properties : (As preventive & curative medicines)

The preventive and curative properties of Rudraksh which have been recorded in the cure of microbial and parasitic infections are as under:-

1. **Anti-viral** : An effective safeguard against all viral infections.
2. **Anti-bacterial** : Protects against all bacterial infections and cures them.
3. **Anti-cancerous** : Effective against the prevention of cancer and also cures it.
4. **Anti-fungal** : A potent safeguard against all pathogenic fungi infections due to them and their cure.
5. **Anti-protozoal** : Both preventive and curative in use against all infections due to parasitic protozoa.
6. **Anti-helminthic** : Effectively preventive and curative against the infections of parasitic helminths and their cure.

Rudraksh Therapy in Ayurvedic System of medicine

As one of the oldest systems of holistic health care, the Indian Science of Ayurveda was founded by the great healer "Bhagwan Dhanwantri". In this perfect science of healing, the underlying principle is based on "creating an energetic balance of the five essential elements in the human body (microcosm) with the five elements of cosmos (macrocosm)." These five elements are : Air, Water, Fire, Sky (Space) and Earth.

A state of balance between the energies of five essential elements of our body with the cosmos maintains a balance and stability in our subtle energy system and also required level of seven essential constituents of human body. These seven constituents are:-

1. Septa Dhatu (liquid)
2. Rakta (blood)
3. Mamsa (flesh)
4. Medha (fat)
5. Asthi (bone)
6. Majja (bone marrow) and
7. Shukra (semen)

In the healing system of the science of Ayurveda, the rudraksh has been described to have high therapeutic properties. Due to the presence of more than one active principle in its chemical composition the rudraksh is frequently used in the treatment of cardiac ailments, mental disorders, convulsions and hypertension.

Ayurveda recommends the use of rudraksh for the health care, well-being of the mankind irrespective of any caste, creed and religion. The therapeutic usage of rudraksh in Ayurveda describes its effective cure in **Tridosha** (defects due to vat, pit & cough) and septadhatus problems related to health. Various medicinal effects of rudraksh described in Ayurveda are as under:-

1. **Kaph, Nashak (Anti-phlegm/anti-mucus):** Due to this property, the rudraskh is an effective remedy against asthma, rhinitis, obesity and endemic health problems.
2. **Vat Nashak : (Anti to excessive gases):** Diseases related to higher level of air/gas element in the body are cured by rudraksh. Some common health problems are :- flatulence, chest and abdominal pain due to excessive gases, headache and rheumatism.

3. **Shirorthi Shamanam (Cure of all head diseases):** All ailments pertaining to eye, ear, nose & throat (EENT) are best cured by rudraksh remedies.
4. **Ruchyam (Cure of stomach ailments):** Rudraksh is used in the cure of indigestion, flatulence, tastelessness and tongue diseases.
5. **Bhutagrah Vishanam (Anti-evil spirit & anti-malefic Planet effects):** Rudraksh not only cures all psychosomatic disorders, harmful effects of evil spirits (possession syndromes and mediumships etc.) but also planetary afflictions.
6. **Aura & Chakra Energizer : (Activator of bio-energetic system of human body):** According to Ayurveda, the holy beads of rudraksh as a part of physical contact therapy maintains and monitors the vibrant flow of bio-cosmic energy in energy chakras and meridians located in human energy system. The optimum flow of energy through our chakra system also regulates a required level of bile, gases (windy air) and phlegm (mucus) in our body. Hence, a perfect balance in health is maintained. Studies have revealed that our healthy chakra system monitors and maintains the energetic level of our aura also. The Aura is a pulsating electromagnetic sheath of bio-energy field around our body and its health is essential for our survival.

Ancient Ayurvedic practitioners recommend that the rosary of fruit of rudraksh is more beneficial than the rosary of beads. It modulates the vital life force (Prantatva or Pran shakti). Besides, it effectively cures mental disorders (unmade) fear and phobia, epilepsy (apasmara), evil effects due to discarnate spirits (Butabadha and pretabadha). The five parts of rudraksh tree called Panchanga (leaves, barks, flowers, fruits and seed) are widely used in Ayurvedic medicine.

The therapeutic properties based on the pharmacological studies on Rudraksh as per Ayurvedic science of medicine are as under–

i. **Rasa** : Amla (Natural Vitamin-C)
ii. **Guna** : Laghu Ruuksha
iii. **Virga** : Ushna (Hot in nature – hence maintains temperature and cardio-vascular circulation of blood)
iv. **Vipaka** : Ushna (Pake ushanam)

v. **Karma** : Ruchya (Curative for stomach ailments, indigestion, flatulence (gas trouble) and tastlessness.

vi. **Dosha Prabhava** : Vatghna (cures problems related to phlegm (mucus) like : asthma, rhinitis, allergies & obesity.

vii. **Vyadhi Prabhava** : (i) Bhuta Grahnasha (Curative for psychosomatic diseases, evil effects and planetary afflictions), (ii) Sirotisamana (Curative for head diseases).

Several experiential and experimental studies have revealed that the rudraksh therapy treatment provides us a perfect healthcare. This system of herbal cure is safer, economical & quick in action for recovery from a disease. In particular, the chronic diseases are well treated with rudraksh therapy as there is no specific and permanent cure of such diseases in the mainstream of western medicines like allopathy.

Four beneficial dimensions which are unique in rudraksh therapy and provide a stable holistic healthcare are as under–

1. **Preventive or Prophylactic in action** : (Resistence against diseases)
2. **Curative in action** (Cures the ailment)
3. **Restorative in action** (Restores the energy of body-mind spirit).
4. **Health maintenance in action** : (Regulates & controls all health factors).

The medicinal system of healing through rudraksh is, therefore, a holistic approach for gaining and maintaining perfect health and well-being of mankind.

A subject survey with regard to frequent use of rudraksh reveals that the following percentage of people and the percentage extent of benefit they get by using rudraksh.

Table : 15

The percentage of people with the percentage of the benefit by using rudraksh

Purpose	Percentage of people	Percentage of Benefit
1. Spiritual gains	30%	50%
2. Relief from Mental Tension	35%	71%
3. Cure for ailments of heart, blood and high blood pressure	35%	85%

Such a subjective survey, therefore, evidently reveals that Rudraksh therapy has more therapeutic value than its spiritual significance.

Modes of Rudraksh Therapy Treatment in Ayurveda

Both external and internal uses of rudraksh in holistic health care and healing program are of multifarious methods which have been described in Ayurveda as under:-

1. **Visual Rudraksh Therapy (VRT)**

   (Rudraksh Dhyan/Darshan chikitsa)

   Just by deep concentration or visual meditation on rudraksh, it enhances bliss and empowerment of the spiritual energy.

Benefits

(1) It improves memory and concentration of thoughts.

(2) It enhances inner peace (bliss) and spiritual energy (empowerment).

Method

(1) Meditation can be exercised on any variety of rudraksh of large size. Rudraksh should be kept in front of your eyes just by hanging it with a string or place it on any object. But in every case, the rudraksh should be at the level of your eyes just in front.

(2) Based on my experiential and experimental knowledge of researches of Rudraksh, I have found the following method of rudraksh meditation much effective:-

Make a figure of OM (ॐ) with rudraksh on any hardboard by using a thin copper wire. Now fix this hardboard on the wall of east side of your room. The level of the board should be in front of your eyes while sitting for meditation facing towards east. Always sit in a pyramid posture.

After you set your sitting posture facing towards east and focus on OM (ॐ) in front of your eyes, just recite 108 times any sacred vibrations (mantras) of your faith/religion. However, to get the best of bliss and peace of mind I have personally found the vibrations of the following mantras more effective. Any of the following two mantras can be adopted for the meditation.

(i) Shiv Om Shiv

(ii) Om Namah Shivaya

2. **Tactual Rudraksh Therapy (TRT)**

Rudraksh sparsh chikitsa or Rudraksh Jap chikitsa)

It is also called 'touch healing Rudraksh therapy'. Physical or contact Rudraksh therapy. The mode of treatment covers the following aspects:-

1. Wearing even a single rudraksh serves as an amulet/ talisman with enormous mystical and medicinal effects. After studding it in silver, it can be worn on arm, ear, head and more commonly just like a necklace around neck with a black thread or any metallic chain.

Researches have revealed that wearing a single rudraksh or its rosary protects the heart-chakra against stressful and inimical vibrations from within the body and also from the damaging effects of accumulated electromagnetic charges of the cosmic field of energy around us. Hence, the use of rudraksh serves as a stress buster, savior of heart and activator of our energy anatomy. By the swinging action of the beads of rudraksh, the negative charges of the body is neutralized and hence, shunted off.

2. Experimental and experiential studies have revealed that a continuous use of rudraksh rosary (mala) gives following benefits–

(1) Cures mental tension, eliminates fear, anxiety, anger, negative thoughts (thinking & attitude).

(2) Cures depression, high blood pressure, sleep and skin disorders.

(3) Enhances will power, self confidence, retentive memory and mental power.

(4) Wearing rudrakh rosary in combination with rosary of beads of Tulsi (*Osimum sanctum*) has been found very effective in the prevention and cure of tuberculosis (T.B.) and respiratory disorders.

3. **Rudraksh Yoga Therapy**

(Rudraksh Yog Sadhana Chikitsa)

Application of Rudraksh sadhana in occult remedies, Yantras, Mantras and Tantra treatments (Kshudra prayogas) has been found to be equally effective in the cure of many psychosomatic diseases and evil spirits, disorders like possession syndrome and mediumship.

4. **Rudraksh Jap Therapy (Counting prayers therapy)**

By counting the holy beads in the rosary of rudraksh between a thumb and a middle finger a natural acupressure influence is exercised in the body which has healing effect. The Jap with rudraksh enhances the power of mind, memory and spiritual energy. The number of beads in a rudraksh rosary should be : 108, 54, 36, 27 and even 18. As far as possible, it should not be less than 27 beads.

5. Rudraksh Acupressure Therapy

The surface of rudraksh has bluntly pointed natural projections which provide excellent acupressure when applied to any specific meridians or acu-points in the body.

I have investigated during my practice that a systematic cyclic movement of rudraksh with pressure on a specific acu-points give remarkable result for the activation of energy chakra and meridians, which in turn cures several ailments. It has been found that the use of rudraksh rosary for jap meditation by pushing the holy beads between finger tips (between thumb and middle finger) activates the most sensitive nerve endings and the energy centres. During this continuous process, a rhythmic natural acupressure influence is exerted which results in the following benefits to the health:

"It improves the blood circulation in eyes, brain, pituitary and pineal gland. It stimulates and monitors the secretion of pineal gland. The stimulation of pineal gland during this process secretes melatonin which is a vital harmone in giving a soothing and blissful condition during meditation (Dhyan prayer). In my personal view, such a type of most effective meditation should preferably be named *Rudra-Acupressure Pulse Meditation*."

6. Medicinal use of Rudraksh for external (local application) and internal (oral) uses:

The medical system of Ayurveda widely recommends the remedies made from herbal rudraksh both for external and internal uses. In the cure of various human ailments, rudraksh is used in the following forms as medicine:-

(1) Rudraksh Powder (Churan)
(2) Rudraksh ashes (Vibhuti or Bhasm)
(3) Rudraksh cold water infusion (Hima)
(4) Rudraksh decoction (for gargling etc.)
(5) Rudraksh oils and emulsions (Tel and Lehyam)
(6) Rudraksh milk
(7) Rudraksh water
(8) Rudraksh paste

(9) Rudraksh eye-drops
(10) Rudraksh injections

Some Important Rudraksh Remedies: Their Preparations and Applications—

(1) Rudraksh Powder (Churan)

Preparation : It is a powder form of rudraksh which can be made by cleaning the rudraksh and grounding it in any grinder as to make a powder of it.

Uses : It is used in making ointments of rudraksh for skin ailments and even for the cure of ulcer. In most of the diseases, the powder of rudraksh is also recommended as an internal medicine.

(2) Rudraksh incinerated ashes (Bhasm or Vibhuti)

Preparation : Best way to make it is to keep some rudraksh beads inside an earthen pot and cover it tightly. Now keep some cakes of cow-dung around this covered earthen pot and burn the dungs. After all the dung turns into ashes, take out the pot and collect the incinerated powdered rudraksh which is called *Bhasm* or *Vibhuti*.

Uses : It is of high medicinal potential and used as an external and internal medicines for the cure of several ailments.

(3) Cold infusion (Hima)

Preparation : It is prepared by infusing rudraksh beads with cold water.

Uses : It cures ailments due to excessive heat and also maintains the metabolism.

(4) Rudraksh decoction (Gargling remedy)

Preparation : Boil any kind of two rudraksh beads in a glass of water for 3 minutes, cool and filter it, the filterate is known as Rudra decoction.

Uses : Gargling with Rudra-decoction cures all oral ailments. It cures mouth sores, ulcer, cracks, and blisters on tongue and in mouth, stomatitis & tastelessness. Such disorders are due to deficiency of Vitamin-C and B_{12} (Riboflavin) which is found in Rudraksh.

(5) Rudraksh oils and emulsions (Til and Lehyam)

Preparation : Put any kind of ten rudraksh beads and nine garlic bulbs in 200ml of gingly oil (Til oil). Boil it for 30 minutes. Now cool and filter this oil. The filterate is called pure Rudraksh oil.

Uses : It is an important remedy for the patients of pneumonia and chest pain. Just apply gently this oil on the chest of the patient and repeat it for 2-3 times a day upto 7 days.

(6) Rudraksh milk

Preparation : Keep any kind of rudraksh (preferably six faced) in a cup of just boiled and slightly cooled milk. Take this milk before going to sleep. Continue taking rudraksh milk for 40 days. Same rudraksh can be reused for forty days after due cleaning to it. However, if it has been boiled in milk, it should not be reused as its medicinal potentials are exhausted after boiling it in milk.

Uses : It cures mental weakness and depletion of memory, loss of memory (amnesia). For smallpox take a two mukhi rudraksh and rub it gently on a clean flat stone, alongwith 2-3 spoons of cow milk. The patient of smallpox should be given this remedial milk paste once a day after meals at night. It should be continued for seven days to cure small-pox.

(7) Rudraksh water

Preparation : Take any kind of rudraksh preferably (five faced) and soak it for over-night in a glass of water which should be kept covered. The rudraksh soaked in water for overnight period becomes fully charged with the active principles in it i.e. called 'Rudraksh water'. My personal studies have found that the use of copper glass or pot yields more effective results due to the addition of copper "ions" in it which are vitally essential for our holistic health.

Uses : (i) Best for the restoration of total health, (ii) Effective for the cure of cardio-vascular diseases, excessive level of lipids and sugar in the blood and also high blood pressure (hypertension), (iii) It empowers the mind 'and memory faculty.

(8) Rudraksh Paste

Preparation : Hold the cone shaped end (upper end) of rudraksh upward and rub its lower end on a hard surface, preferably a flat stone. Add little water or milk to it to make a paste of it.

Uses : It is best for licking as an internal medicine. For the cure of hyper-acidity and stomatitis, it is also used in the cure of various types of skin infections when applied locally on skin.

(9) Rudraksh eye-drops

Preparation : A clean rudraksh should be kept in rose water or distilled water for 3-4 hours. This water can be used as medicinal eye-drop.

Uses : It cures conjunctivitis and also improves the eye-sight.

(10) Rudraksh injections

Preparation : Some pharmaceutical companies in Belgium have patented the Rudraksh injections. These injections which contain the concentrate of the active principles found in rudraksh have been found very effective in the treatment of cardio-vascular diseases.

Uses : Studies have revealed that these injections strengthen the heart and will-power of a person and also keep away the disorders of depression, high-blood pressure and heart attack.

Cure of some specific diseases through Rudraksh remedies

Some specific diseases and their cure with rudraksh therapy have been reported as under:-

1. Diseases of Nervous system and sense organs.
2. Diseases of mouth, throat and digestive system.
3. Diseases of heart and blood vascular system.
4. Diseases of respiratory system.
5. Diseases of kidney.
6. Diseases of skin and hair.
7. Diseases of reproductive system.
8. Diseases of bones and joints.

General Diseases

1. Immunity disorders.
2. Cure of venomous bites by scorpion & insects.

Diseases of Nervous System and Sense organs:

(1) Nervous Numbness:

Remedy : (i) Mix rudraksh powder in a spoonful of honey and take it daily with milk for 40 days, (ii) Rudraksh ash (Vibhuti bhasm) when smeared on the body, gives warming effect and cures numbness.

Benefit : It invigorates nervous system and cures numbness of the body.

(2) General weakness

Remedy : Two grams of rudraksh powder mixed with honey should be taken daily after meals for 80 days. It is very effective and general tonic for the body.

Benefit : Best for total health and used as a general tonic.

(3) Mental weakness (mind & memory weakness)

Remedy : Before going to sleep, keep a four or six faced rudraksh in just boiled milk, lukewarm it and take this milk for 21 to 40 days regularly.

Benefit : It is best for increasing the concentration of mind and memory power.

(4) Insomnia (sleeplessness)

Remedy : Mix one gram of rudraksh Bhasm with one gram of Swarnamakshik bhasm and take it twice with butter for 21 days. Hot food, drinks should be avoided during the course of treatment.

Benefit : Insomnia is permanently cured through this remedy.

5. Headache

Remedy : Mix in equal parts the rudraksh powder and dry ginger powder and make a paste of it with water. Apply this paste on the forehead for one hour and wash thereafter with lukewarm water.

Benefit : It is quick and effective permanent treatment for various types of headache including migraine.

6. Epilepsy & Delirium

Remedy : (i) Mix one gram of rudraksh churan with 2 gram of saraswathi churan. It should be taken 2 times a day for 90 days. Hot and non-vegetarian foods should be avoided during the course of treatment.

(ii) Take a six mukhi rudraksh, rub it on a flat clean stone with 2-3 spoonful of water and make a thin paste of it. Apply this paste on forehead for 21 days.

(iii) A teaspoonful pulp of rudraksh should be taken with water for 7 days.

Benefit : It gives complete cure of epilepsy and delirium ailments.

7. Possession syndrome and evil spirit afflictions

Remedy : Wear either of 4, 5, 6 faced rudraksh on full moon (Poornima) or new moon (Amavasya) after due ritual of its purification and activation.

Benefit : It cures evil spirits, afflictions and possession syndrome problems related to health.

(8) Bad Dreams

Remedy : A preventive remedy to keep away any kind of bad dreams is to keep any type of rudraksh under your pillow during sleep.

Benefit : It will stop the problems of bad dreams, fear and phobia.

(9) Nervous debility (weakness of nerves & brain)

Remedy : Mix equal quantity of rudraksh powder with pear bhasm and two grams of coral bhasm. It should be taken once a day for 30 days.

Benefit : It causes general weakness of nerve & brain.

Diseases of Sense Organs

Diseases of eyes

(10) Eye-sight weakness and cataract

Remedy : A three faced rudraksh should be at first thoroughly washed in clean water then rubbed in milk and applied to the eyes like kajal.

Benefit : It improves the eye-sight and cures cataract within 15 to 30 days.

Exercise : See the early sunrise constantly for five minutes through a rosary of Rudraksh and also touch it to the eye-lids after every seeing. This nature cure exercise should be repeated for 80 days.

(11) Conjunctivitis and burning sensation of eyes

Remedy : Take any facial variety of rudraksh (preferably five faced), clean it and keep it in rose water for 4 hours and then decant the rose water. The decanted rose water becomes an effective eye-drop. This rudraksh eye-drop should be used as 1-2 drops daily in the eyes for 2-3 days.

Diseases of ear

(12) Hard of hearing/paracusis

Remedy : Boil any kind of rudraksh in a half cup of mustard (sarson) oil, cool it and decant it. Put 2 drops of soil in the ear for 3 days.

Benefit : It softens the wax of the ear and cures inner inflammation and also paracusis/hard of hearing.

Diseases of mouth, throat & digestive

(13) Stomatitis (Inflamation inside mouth)

Remedy : Gargling with rudraksh decocation 2 times a day for 3-4 days cures stomatitis.

Benefit : Rudraksh has rich content of vitamin-C and B_{12}. It cures stomatitis and even the ulcerative conditions for which the treatment duration should be prolonged for 7 to 10 days.

(14) Inflammation and cracks in tongue

Remedy : Purify some beads of clean and dried rudraksh by soaking them in coconut water for 24 hours and ground them into powder, now take two grams of this powder and half gram of coral bhasm, now mix them in honey. Apply this paste on tongue 2 times a day for 21 days. Nothing should be taken for 30 minute after applying this medicine on the tongue. For quick and best results, gargling with rudraksh decoction should also be done 2 times a day.

Benefit : This treatment cures inflammation and cracks on the tongues which are associated with tastelessness, numbness and burning sensation.

(15) Stammering of voice

Remedy : (i) Put 2 beads of four mukhi rudraksh in a cup of just boiled milk. On cooling, remove the rudraksh and take the milk. It should be repeated for 90 days. Rudraksh beads taken out of milk should be washed properly with water dried and kept safely for reuse.

(ii) Mix rudraksh powder with Akkalkarra powder in honey and rub it on tongue 2-3 times a day. It improves the tone of the voice and makes it sharp and vibrant.

Benefit : It cures all stammering conditions of the tongue and voice.

(16) Tonsils and other throat diseases

Remedy : A rudraksh rosary (Necklace or Kantmala) just tied around the base of the neck cures tonsils and other ailments of the throat disease including the breathing disorders due to chest congestion.

Benefit : It is an effective treatment for the cure of throat diseases.

(17) Indigestion, Nausea and vomiting:

Remedy (i) : Take any kind of rudraksh (preferably 14 mukhi) clean and dry it. Now keep it in a cup of ordinary water for five minutes. Take this rudraksh water 2-3 times a day.

For chronic indigestion, take a teaspoonful powder of rudraksh of any type and mix equal quantity of pepper powder and make a dose of this mixture.

(18) Constipation

Remedy (i): At night, keep any kind of rudraksh in a copper glass filled with water. Cover the glass and keep it overnight. By morning, the water gets fully charged with the ions of copper with rudraksh. It is called 'Copper ion rudraksh water'. This water should be taken early in the morning, preferably empty stomach.

My investigations have revealed that along with rudraksh if a coin of pure silver or rod of pure silver is also immersed in water for overnight period, it gives much effective results and this medicinal water is called 'copper-silver ion rudra-water'.

Benefit : It cures constipation effectively and also best for total health, if taken regularly. It also cures stomach pain due to indigestion, loose motion and gas trouble.

Remedy (ii) : Mix rudraksh paste with ginger juice and take one spoonful of it daily for 3 to 5 days. Another remedy includes mixing the pulp of rudraksh fruit with swaras of vasa and tulsi. Keep them mixed in a kharal of one night. Take one spoonful of it 2 times a day.

Benefit : It cures indigestion, flatulence, loss of appetite and loose motion.

Diseases of Heart and Blood Vascular System

(19) High Blood Pressure

Remedy (i) : Wearing any kind of rudraksh against heart chakra not only protects heart but also controls and regulates the high blood pressure. Hence, this Rudraksh remedy is both preventive and curative in action.

My concurrent investigations have established that rudraksh wearing removes from the body all static bio-electrical impulses and regulates the optimum flow of positive impulses in the blood circulation. This prevents heart attack. Studies have revealed that rudraksh absorbs excessive heat of the body and releases it to outside, hence it serves as a heat filter for the body as a thermo-regulatory remedy. So, the wearing of rudraksh protects us from excessive rise in body temperature and related harmful effects.

Remedy (ii) A single dose of one ratti 250 mg. bhasm of rudraksh is most effective in the control and cure of high blood pressure. It should be taken with milk or curd for at least 7days. My personal observations have found that a dose of one ratti rudraksh bhasm mixed with 1 ratti gold bhasm (swarn Bhasm) if taken with milk/curd for 7days, it gives magical results in the treatment of hypertension and mental anxiety.

Remedy (iii) In order to control higher fluctuations of blood-pressure, wear 16 beads of five faced rudraksh on each arm; 12 beads of rudraksh on wrist and 108 beads of rudraksh on chest region which must touch the heart level.

(20) Cure for all diseases of heart and cardiovascular system

Remedy (i) : Rudraksh water medication gives total healthcare to the heart and cardio-vascular system. Take any kind of a rudraksh preferably 5 faced, clean it and put it in a copper glass filled with water. Now cover the glass and keep it soaked in water for the over-night. By morning the water becomes fully charged with the ions of copper. This medicinal water should be taken empty stomach every morning. The same rudraksh can be used for 40 days. However, it should not be reused after 40 days because its medicinal potentials are exhausted.

Benefit : This remedy is effective in the cure of all ailments of heart and blood circulation.

Remedy (ii) Rudraksh garlic-water is another effective remedy for the total care of heart and cure of different ailments of the cardio-vascular system. So, three beads of rudraksh and one garlic-piece (bulb) in a glass of water should be kept covered overnight. Take this medicinal water early in the morning for 60 days.

Benefit : It is most effective for the cure of hypertension and the disorders associated with the function of heart.

Remedy (iii) Rudraksh garlic-milk is equally effective for the total care and cure of heart. Boil in a cup of milk a rudraksh of any face alongwith one bulb of garlic. This medicinal milk is effective for the control of higher level of cholesterol. It should be taken for 3 months. My observations have revealed that the milk soaked garlic bulb in this treatment should also be consumed alongwith the rudraksh garlic milk.

Benefit : It is a remarkable anti-cholesterol remedy which is both preventive and curative to the ailments of heart and blood circulation. It keeps away the risks of heart attack which is fatal to life.

Remedy (iv) Rudraksh honey tonic should be prepared by mixing some powder of rudraksh with honey. One teaspoonful of this honey should be taken daily after meals for 80 days.

Benefit : It is a general cardio-vascular tonic and also enhances the vigour and vitality of the body.

Remedy (v) Rudraksh rosary which touches the level of heart not only cures but also serves as an effective remedy for the ailments of heart. The rosary of rudraksh should be long enough to touch the level of heart. It also enhances the strength of heart muscles for its total health.

Benefit : It energies the heart chakra for its total health.

Diseases of Respiratory system

(21) Whooping cough

Remedy (i) : Take any kind of rudraksh preferably 10 mukhi and rub it on any flat stony surface alongwith 1 table spoonful of milk. The medicinal extract prepared as such should be taken three times a day as under :

One table spoon in the morning (empty stomach);

One table spoon in the day time (after lunch);

One table spoon at night (after dinner).

(ii) Mix equal parts of the powder of five faced rudraksh and the powder of stem of tulsi in honey. Take this medicine one spoonful daily.

Benefit : It cures chronic cough (Phlegm cough) and gives soothing relief to the patient.

(22) Asthma, Bronchitis and Spastic pain

Remedy : Mix one gram of rudraksh powder with honey. Take one teaspoonful two times a day. It is anti-phlegm hence, cures chest congestion due to mucus. It is best for children.

(23) Pneumonia

Remedy : The medicine prescribed above for asthma should be given 3 times a day. The spastic chest pain due to pneumonia and other respiratory disorders can be cured by applying lukewarm rudraksh oil for 2-3 times a day. This oil can be prepared as under:

Boil any kind of ten rudraksh in 200 ml. of gingerly oil (Til oil) for 30 minutes and filter the oil. The Filterate is called rudraksh oil.

Diseases of Kidney and Urinary Tract Infection (U.T.I.)

(24) Nephritis (Dysfunction of kidney) & UTI:

Remedy : Tie with a copper wire five beads of five faced rudraksh. Keep this device for overnight in a cleaned copper jug containing 4 glasses of water. On next day, the patient should take this medicinal water four times a day. One glass should be taken early in the morning before breakfast, one glass of water after lunch, one after dinner and one at bed time. This remedial treatment should be continued for 40 days. Every day fill the copper jug with four glasses of water and take them in the next day.

Benefit : It is best remedy not only for the permanent cure of nephritis but also prevents further relapse of the disease.

Diseases of skin and hair

(25) Leucoderma

Remedy (i) Mix some bhasm of nine or five faced rudraksh with the extract of tulsi leaves and make a paste of it. Just apply thin paste on the affected parts of the body for 3 months.

(ii) Mix some bhasm of nine or five mukhi rudraksh with the ground powder of the roots of tulsi plant. Make a paste of it in a clean water or Gangajal and apply it on the affected parts due to leucoderma.

Benefit : The patches of leucoderma will dry up and vanish with this treatment.

(26) Itch, Eczema & Pimples:

Remedy (i) : Grind some leaves of neem tree (Margosa) with rudraksh powder and make a thin paste of it with water. Apply this paste on the affected area of the skin for two times a day.

(ii) Mix some bhasm of 5 faced rudraksh with the dried & powder dung of black cow. Make a thin paste of it in Gangajal or distilled water. Apply this paste on the affected area of the skin.

Benefit : It cures all chronic ailments of the skin. It is most effective in curing the skin problems like itch, eczema & pimples.

(27) Facial spots, black marks and blemishes

Remedy (i) : Mix some powder of five faced rudraksh with some extract of tulsi leaves (*ocimum sanctum,*) and add some lemon juice to it. Apply this paste on the affected area of the face for 7 days.

(ii) Mix some rudraksh powder with fresh lime juice and sandal wood powder to make a paste of it in water. Now apply this paste on the affected area of the face. Keep the smear of the paste at least for an hour and wash it with lukewarm water. For best results, apply this paste at night and remove it in the morning by using lukewarm water.

Benefit : It is an effective cure for blemishes, black marks and other facial spots. It gives glamour and glow to the face.

(28) Special wrinkles and dullness of facial skin

Remedy : Take some rudraksh powder preferably 8 faced. Mix it with almond and rose water to make a paste of it. Smear this thin paste on the face and dry it for about one hour. Repeat this remedy for seven days.

Benefit : This treatment nourishes the skin and enhances its glow, glamour and sensitivity.

(29) Skin Inflammation

Remedy : Make a paste of rudraksh powder in the urine of cow. Lukewarm it and apply the same to the affected area due to inflammation.

Benefit : It gives instant relief from the painful inflammatory conditions of the skin.

(30) Skin Burns and Scalds

Remedy : Mix some powder of 5 faced rudraksh in coconut oil and also add some camphor to it. Now anoint or smear this ointment on the burn affected area.

Benefit : It is effective in the healing of wounds and also does not allow the growth of secondary infection.

(31) Scar due to Burn / Wound

Remedy : Just place any faced variety of rudraksh on a scar and fix it with an adhesive tape on the scar for overnight period. Remove the tape in the morning then rub it with lemon juice on it. Now again put the tape in the same way and next day also and repeat this exercise for seven days.

Benefit : It absorbs all marks or scar due to skin diseases, wounds and burns etc. It also regenerates the growth of skin pigment called melanin.

Diseases of Hair

(32) Greying of Hair

Remedy : Make a paste of the powder of rudraksh with the extract of fresh Amla. Now apply this paste at the roots of graying hair once a day. It should be applied during night and the hair should be washed with lukewarm water in the morning for much better results. This treatment should be continued for 90 days.

Benefit : This treatment not only stops the greying of hair but also enhances their growth.

(33) Falling of Hair and Baldness

Remedy : Make a paste of powder of some rudraksh (10 faced) preferably) with the extract of some fresh tender leaves of Neem tree (Margosa). Now apply this paste on the affected parts for the 3 months.

Benefit : This treatment is best both for partial and complete loss of hair (Alopacea). It stops the loss of hair and also increases the growth of hair effectively.

Diseases of reproductive system

(34) Gonorrhoea

Remedy (i) : The four faced rudraksh should be kept for the overnight period in a copper glass full of water. Take this copper ion water early in the morning empty stomach and repeat it for 21 days. For much better results, a 4 faced rudraksh studded with silver should be worn as pendant.

(ii) Silver pendant of 4 faced rudraksh should be worn with a black thread around neck. This remedy enhances the effectivity of results.

Benefit : It prevents and cures Gonorrhoea infection. It also gives satisfactory relief to the patient.

(35) Impotency

Remedy : Make a paste of any facial variety of rudraksh by rubbing it with water on a flat stony surface. Apply this paste on the forehead once a day. It should be repeated for 90 days.

Benefit : It improves sexual power and cures impotency.

(36) Frigidity of Female

The above cited paste should be applied by the female on the nipple of her breast for 21 days. It cures frigidity.

Benefit : This remedy is most effective in enhancing the sexual urge in females and relieves them from frigidity problem.

Diseases of bones and joints

(37) Arthritis and Rheumatism

Remedy : Take a rudraksh of any face clean it and boil it in a glass of goat milk. Now take out the rudraksh from the milk, lukewarm it and take it daily for 21 days.

Benefit : It is very effective remedy for arthritis and rheumatism.

(38) Backache and waist pain

Remedy : Belt of any facial variety of rudraksh should be used around waist for 21 days. It can be removed during night. A belt must contain as many as 108 beads of rudraksh.

Benefit : It is preventive and curative for backache and waist pain. For better results, a rosary of rudraksh with 51 beads should be worn around the neck.

(39) Rheumatic arthritis

Remedy : Take two grams of powder of the pulp of rudraksh fruit. Mix it with 3 grams of powder of Vivili leaves. This medicine should be taken 2 times a day with water and should be continued for 7 to 40 days depending upon the severity of the problem.

For best results also, use a local application of paste made from mixing two parts of rudraksh powder (any variety) in milk butter cream and 2 parts of pepper, one part of pippali. This paste should be applied once a day on the affective area.

Benefit : It cures Rheumatic arthritis and typhoid fever.

Rudraksh remedy for the cure of serious health problems due to immunity deficiency

(40) Immunity deficiency diseases

Remedy : Wearing of rudraksh of any facial variety maximizes the immunity. It is the source of Vitamin-C for a patient. It prevents and cures all immune deficiency diseases like AIDS, cancer etc. Studies have revealed that regular use of rudraksh as rosary and also by taking rudraksh water strengthens the entire neuro immuno-complex of the body. It serves as a sentinel against the erosion of the immunity of a living system.

(41) Rudraksh prescription for cancer

Remedy : Concurrent experiential studies have revealed that a special type of rudraksh known as 'Amlasar Rudraksh' is very effective in the cure of cancer. It should be rubbed in cow milk and an extract of one spoonful of it should be taken once a day after meals. Amlasar Rudraksh is a special variety of rudraksh which is round in shape but without any furrow on it. It is also called a streakless variety of rudraksh like the Amla (*Emblica officinalis*). It is green in colour and found mainly in Kashi, Pithoragarh and Chamoli areas of India.

Benefit : It has a magical cure for cancer.

(42) Small pox and chicken pox infections:

Remedy: (i) Take a two faced rudraksh, rub it gently on clean flat stone alongwith 2-3 spoons of cow milk. The patient of the smallpox should lick this remedial milk once in a day. It should be continued for seven days.

(ii) Mix equal quantity of the powder of 5 faced rudraksh with the powder of neem bark and make their well mixed paste in honey. Take one spoonful of this medicine daily thrice a day.

Benefit : It is effective cure both for small pox and chicken pox.

General prescriptions of Rudraksh

(43) Cholera infection:

Remedy: (i) A necklace made from the string of copper wire rudraksh seeds and papaya seeds should be worn around neck for 40 days.

(ii) For better results, equal number of some seeds of rudraksh and papaya should be used together in a single pendant type made copper encasement. It should be worn like a necklace with black thread.

Benefit : It is effective for the cure of Cholera and also prevents this infection.

(44) Stings of scorpions and insects:

Remedy : Rub a five faced rudraksh on a grind stone, with the fresh juice of lemon and apply this paste on the affected parts of the body due to bite/stings of insects or scorpions.

Benefit : This treatment subsides the pain due to stings and bites of all arthropods and also cures them by preventing the secondary infection.

Section IV

GUEST CONTRIBUTIONS FROM EXPERTS

Chapter 8

Rudraksha : The power Beads of India

❑ **Prof. G.S. Lavekar**

Rudraksha (*Elaeocarpus sphaericus* (Gaertn.) K. Schum) syn. *E. ganitrus* Roxb; *Ganitrus sphaericus* Gaertn.

Family : Elaeocarpaceae.

Introduction

Rudraksha are the dried seeds of the fruits obtained from the tree *Elaeocarpus sphaericus* (Gaertn.) K. Schum., which grows in the selected locations of South Asia i.e. Northern India and Nepal and South East Asia (Java, Korea and parts of Malaysia, Taiwan and China) and known as "Ultrasum-bead tree and '*Blue marble tree*' in English and *Rudraksha* in Sanskrit, Tamil, Telugu, Kannada and Marathi and *Rudraki* in Hindi, *Rudrakhya* in Bengali, *Rudrakhyo* in Oriya and *Rudraio* in Assam.

Distribution

In India about 25 species of *Elaeocarpus* are found. Rudraksha tree (*Elaeocarpus sphaericus*) commonly occurs in the foothills of all districts of Arunachal Pradesh, Bhutan and Sikkim, West Bengal, Bihar, Madhya Pradesh and Maharashtra. Rudraksha trees are found in tropical ever green forests which are characterized by three tier forest stands and it is usually present in the second stand.

Description

Elaeocarpus is a medium to large sized tree and occasionally cultivated as an ornamental tree. Leaves are oblong-lanceolate, sub-entire and smooth. Flowers are white in colour and found in dense racemes arising mostly from old leaf axils. Fruit is bluish purple coloured drupe which is globose or obovoid (3.40 mm:1/8 to 1 ½ inches) enclosing a hard, longitudinally grooved, tubercled, normally 5-celled stone (seed). The fruit has smooth light green skin and pulp much like a green grape.

Power Beads

The stones are used to be cleared, polished, sometimes stained and then used as beads for rosaries, bracelets and other spiritual jewelry used to be ornamental objects setting in gold or silver and is known as power beads of India for its unique power to gain calmness of the mind for only individual. Rudraksha beads were used to instill for the calmness in mind, intellectual pursuits and had powers to cleanse all the 7 vital chakras in the human body. One should use those rudraksha only which are strong, well thorny, clearly grooved facets and with natural self-holed.

Origin of Rudraksha

The word rudraksha, in fact, comes from the two Sanskrit words *rudra*, synonym for *Lord Shiva*, and *aksha*, meaning "eyes", which means tears of Siva. In India, the miraculous and medicinal powers of Rudraksha beads were known since 5000 BC. Yogis and Adepts of India have worn Rudraksh beads for thousands of years because of its ability to enhance *meditation practice and control of mind.* In ancient India, vast amount of Vedic literature was to be studied and memorized by students. According to the Siva Purana, for the sake of world peace, Lord Siva sat in meditation for 1000 years with his eyes closed and when he opened his eyes, a few drops of tear fell to the ground and became the holy Rudraksha tree, whose seeds have become an *emblem for spiritual austerity and power.* It is considered as spiritual power beads of India. One who wears the rudraksha in the prescribed manner will invoke the energies of Lord Shiva and negative thoughts and emotions will be destroyed. In various ancient scriptures (i.e. Padma Purana, Shiva Purana, Mantramaharnava, Rudrajabalopanishad) it is proclaimed that if a person meets his death while wearing a rudraksha he is released from the cycle of life and death and achieves moksha (libertation).

Therapeutic Use

रुद्राक्षमम्लमुष्णज्यवातध्नं कफनाशनम्।
षिरोत्तिषमनं रुच्यं भूतग्रहविनाशनम्।।

(राजनिघन्टू)

It is *amla* (sour) ushna (hot), pacifies vitiated vata and kapha; relieves headache; an appetizer and beneficial in mental diseases and epileptic fits (Rajnighatu).

Prof. P.V. Sharma (Dravyya Guna Vigyan, 1983) mentioned that the fruit (seeds kernel) is sweet, cooling, ambient, sedative, expectorant and antipyretic and is useful in epileptic fits, melancholia, maniac conditions, convulsions and vitiated conditions of kapha and vata.

According to Ayurveda, Rudraksha contains more natural vitamin C which increases the immunity against any disease. Rudraksha is hot in nature, hence it helps in proper blood circulation, equal distribution of energy to all the parts of human body and melts out the excess quantity of cholesterol in the blood and thus keep the heart ailments away. It is *Vataghana*, hence Rudraksha plays a vital role in treating chest pain and early stages of rheumatic pain. It is also *kuphanashak* and helpful in obesity and unwanted over swelling etc. Rudraksha is *Ruchyam* which means it is used to enhance the taste.

On the basis of pharmacological experiments made by Indian and foreign experts it is proved that Rudraksha shows the following biological activities.

1. Anti-bacterial
2. Anti-fungal
3. Anti-protozoal
4. Anti-helmintic
5. Anti-viral and
6. Anti-cancer properties (Sathyanarayana Swamy K.2000)

Chemical Constituents

Fruits contain palmitic, linoleic and myristic acids, from the leave some alkaloids are reported i.e. (-) auoclacocarpilize, clacocarpidine, alelcocarpus (-) epiabelaeocarpiline and others (Ashima Chatterjee, 1994).

Pharmacology

Pharmacological investigations with the water soluble portion of 90% ethanol extract of the fruits of *Elaeocarpus sphaericus* showed the presence of a prominent central nervous system depressant effect, characterized behavioural, actions potentialion of hexobarbitone hypnosis and morphine analgesia, anti-convulsant and anti-amphetamine effects. In addition the extract showed a cardio-stimulant, depressor, smooth musclę relaxant and hydrocholeretic activities, part of these being mediated through beta adrenoreceptor stimulation and in part through a direct musculotropic effect. The pharmacological profile of activity of the extract substantiates the use of the plant fruits in the treatment of mental diseases, epilepsy, hypertension, asthma and liver diseases in the ancient Indian systems of medicine (Bhattacharya S.K., 1975).

Anti-bacterial Activity

Anti-bacterial activity of petroleum ether benzenes, chloroform, acetone and ethanol, extracts of dried Elaeocarpus sphaericus fruit was investigated against gram positive and gram negative bacteria using disc diffusion and plate dilution methods. It is observed that alkaloids and flavonoids present in the fruit appear to be of chemotherapeutic interest. The Acetone fraction showed marked anti-microbial activity against ten organisms. Benzene was active against *Salmonella typhimurium* and *Morganella morganii*, and Ethanol against *Plesiomonas shigelloides*, *Shigella flexnerii* and *Shigella sosonneii* (R.K. Singh and Gopal Nath, 1999).

Anti-inflammatory activity

Sequential petroleum ether, benzene, chloroform, acetone and ethanol extracts (50-200 or 200 mg./kg., ip, or 200 mg./kg. po) of dried fruits of Rudraksha, pretreatment time 30-45 min. showed significant anti-inflammatory activity against both acute and sub-acute models, analgesic barbiturate-hypnosis potentialion and antiulcerogenic activities in rats. All the extracts except petroleum ether and ethanol decreased swim stress immobility in mice indicating some degree of antidepressant activity. All the extracts protected guinea-pigs against bronchospams induced by histamine and acetycholine aerosols. Chemically, the extracts showed the presence of glycosides, steroids, alkaloids and flavnoids (R.K. Singh, et.al., 2000).

Rudraksha Therapy

Rudraksha therapy is also well known in China and Japan. In Chinese tradition it is believed that most of the illness is caused due to improper balancing of **Yin & Yang** and disruption in the flow of **Chi** energy. Rudraksha were considered to enhance the flow of **Chi** – the life energy in the body and thus the balance of **Yin & Yang** is maintained. In Japan, the Rudraksha beads were widely used in Zen Buddhist sector for meditation which was taken to Japan by Buddhist monks from India.

There is a strong belief that, merely on holding the Rudraksha beads in hand or wearing them even for few hours one can very clearly feel the heightened energy levels. Every one who wore the Rudraksha beads found benefits in enhanced pace of mind, tranquility, better health, success and prosperity and good luck factor enabling one to achieve many things hitherto considered impossible. Rudraksha has potent anti-aging properties.

Rudraksha mala mainly consists of 108 beads and they are usually found with five sections, or faces, built can occur from one to 22 faces. There are an additional 16 types of Rudraksha with unusual shapes and configurations. There are various qualities attributed to the number of face and shapes found in a Rudraksha bead which are as follows:

- **1 Face :** (Rarest) For the Sun and Lord Siva. Spiritual liberation and attainment of all material desires, including power, authority, wealth, and all comforts of life. Eradication of all troubles & problems, attainment of peace of mind, true happiness and success.

  Mantra : Om Namah Sivaya. Om Hreem Namaha.
- **2 Faces** : (Rare) For the Moon, Devi, Ardhanarishvara and Gaurishankar, good for diseases of the left eye, kidney, stomach. Improves human relationships, promotes sattwic qualities, increases spiritual power, concentration, peace of mind, and happiness.

  Mantra : Shree Gauri Shankaraya Namaha. Om Namaha.
- **3 Faces** : (Rare) For Mars and Agni, the Fire God. For purification of sins and mastery over the three worlds-gross, mental, spiritual. Good for blood disorders, physical weakness, menstrual disorders, fear, doubt, guilt,

depression, inferiority complex, litigation, protection against vehicle accidents, and snake bites.

Mantra : Om Kleem Namah.

- **Faces** : (Unusual) For Mercury and Lord Brahma. Good for clear thinking, intelligence, speech, logic, creativity, communication skills, and memory.

  Mantra : Om Hreem Namaha.

- **5 Faces :** (Most common) For Jupiter, Pancha Brahma, Kalagni Rudra. Smaller beads good for meditation and japa. Good for blood circulation, cardiovascular health, schizophrenia, manic depression, poverty. Attracts divine grace, promotes positive thinking, mental peace, fulfilment of all desires, and spiritual protection.

  Mantra : Om Hreem Namaha.

- **6 Faces** : For Venus, Ganesha, and Kartikeya/ Subrahmanian. Good for love, romance, relationships, music, fine arts, creative expression, problems with throat and reproductive organs, fainting and hysteria. Gives steady mind, intelligence, wisdom, and success in business, education and examinations, and achievement of all comforts of life.

  Mantra : Om Hreem Hum Namaha. Swami Kaartikeya Namaha.

- **7 Faces** : For Saturn, Sapta Rishi, Manmadan, and Mahalakshmi. Protects against old age, disease, death, impotence, poor circulation, hopelessness, despair, delays, obstructions, scarcity, worry. Helps one to attain respect, prosperity, spiritual power, and material success.

  Mantra : Om Hum Namaha. Om Mahalakshmi Namaha.

- **8 Faces** : For Rahu (ascending lunar node), Bhairava, and Ganesha. Good for overcoming all obstacles to material success and achievement of all worldly goals.

  Mantra : Om Hum Namaha. Om Ganeshaya Namaha.

- **9 Faces** : For Ketu (descending lunar node), Goddess Durga, Bhairava, and Kapil Muni. Good for protection against misfortunes, black magic, miscarriage, low energy, ennui, dissipative outlook, lack of inspiration. Gives energy to materialize one's desires (kriyashakti) as well as to progress on the spiritual path.

  Mantra : Nava Durgayi Namaha. Om Hreem Hum Namaha.

- **10 Faces** : For 10 Avatars of Lord Vishnu, Protection in the 10 directions. Gives overall protection from all planetary influences, protection from spirits and black magic, security and self-confidence. Family is protected for many generations.
  Mantra : Shree Narayanaaye Namaha. Shree Vishnavai Namaha. Om Hreem Namaha.
- **11 Faces** : (Very Rare) For Lord Indra, Ekadasa Rudra, and Lord Hanuman. Gives exceptional courage, strength, power, energy, charisma, adventurous spirit and daring. Helps women to attract and protect an auspicious husband. Wisdom, success, good judgment, protection from accidents.
  Mantra : Om Shree Rudraya Namaha. Om Hreem Num Namaha.
- **12 Faces** : For the Sun God, Surya, and Lord Vishnu. Attracts all Divine blessings, removes obstacles and worries. Protects against enemies and accidents. Increases leadership and executive abilities, radiance, and strength. Good for diseases of right eye, headache, ear ailments, bone weakness; lack of confidence, charisma, personal power.
  Mantra : Shree Suryaya Namaha.
- **13 Faces** : For Lord Indra, Kamadeva, Shanmuganatha, and Vishwadevas. Gives attainment and enjoyment of all worldly desires, good health, prosperity, honor, love, intelligence, spiritual power and Divine wisdom.
  Mantra : Om Hreem Namaha.
- **14 Faces** : (Very Rare) For Lord Siva and Hanuman. Activates third eye chakra for higher clairvoyance, intuitive perception, correct decision making. Cures diseases, bestows all comforts and luxuries of life, and a high position of power and authority.
  Mantra : Om Namah Sivaya.
- **15 Faces** : (Very Rare) For Pashupati. Activates clairvoyance and gives increased energy to materialize all desires. Promotes good health, spiritual power, and prosperity for entire family. Elevates soul and blesses one with happiness, inner peace, and fulfilment of life purpose. Protects against skin diseases.
  This type is found to be very ideal in ventures, speculation like stock markets. In ancient Indian mythology, there

have been various instances of kings and aristocracy using these types of Rudraksha beads for success in gaming, speculative activity and future predictions.

- **16 Faces** : (Very Rare) Worn by ascetics living in jungles for protection against heat and cold. Keep on puja altar for prosperity to entire family.
- **17 Faces** : (Very Rare) For Viswakarma. Attracts prosperity, wealth, property, vehicles.
- **18 Faces** : (Very Rare) For Bhu mata – Mother Earth. For happiness, good health, and protection of children.
- **19 Faces** : For Narayanaya. Attainment of all worldly pleasures.
- **20 Faces** : For Brahmans. For continued protection of spiritual practice.
- **21 Faces** : For Kubera, God of Wealth. For unimaginable wealth.

Gauri-Shankar (two beads joined together naturally) : (Very Rare) Supports harmony and integration of male and female energies. Helps attract soul mate or life partner, and brings happiness in marriage.

Mantra : Om Gaurishankaraya Namaha.

Ganesh Rudraksha : (Rudraksha with protusion like the trunk of Ganesha) Perfection in every area of life.

Ganesh-Gauri (one small and one larger bead naturally joined together): (Very rare) Good for having children.

How to use and care for the Rudraksha mala

- It is best to wear the rudraksha mala for the first time on a Monday. If at all possible, it should be first brought to a Shiva temple for sanctification early on a Monday morning and then worn immediately after worship. If a Shiva temple is not available then simply wear it initially on a Monday.
- At bedtime, remove the mala and place it on any alternate place of your home. When traveling, you should sleep with it on.
- After bathing in the morning hold the mala in the right hand and repeat the appropriate mantra for 108 times.
- Do not wear the rudraksha mala during period of menstrual bleeding or while attending funerals.
- The rudraksha mala has a very long life span. A properly cared for mala can be passed along to eight generations as a family heirloom.

- The rudraksha mala can be washed occasionally with warm soapy water and allowed to dry naturally.

Some of the different aspects where Rudraksha therapy is ideal are:

1. **Mind related** : Like stress, depression, mood disorders, lack of concentration, feelings of not being in control.
2. **Physical level** : Like blood pressure high and low, cardiac ailments, breathing troubles, asthma, heart troubles. Effects enhanced stamina and energy levels, boosts immune system.
3. **Spiritual level** : Rudraksha beads are very ideal for Meditation, enhanced state of awareness, reiki, excellent peace of mind, feeling of well-being in tune with nature and the infinite intelligence and Yoga practice.

Rudraksha Therapy may be carried out by 4 fold methods:

i) Darshan (By touch and inhalation)

a. By wearing Rudraksha Mala
b. By doing Japa (Chanting of Mantras) with Rudraksha.
c. By Rudraksha Dhoopam (Fumigation).
d. Rubbing on Rudraksha beads (Acupressure) having Magnet inside.

ii) Sevana

a. Rudraksha Churan (Powder)
b. Rudraksha water Hima (cold infusion)
c. Rudraksha decoction for gargling
d. Rudraksha milk
e. Rudraksha Bhasma/Vibhuti
f. Rudraksha oil
g. Rudraksha Leham (Jam)
h. Rudraksha eye drops
i. Rudraksha paste

iii) Yoga Sadhana

a. Rudraksha Mandep
b. Rudraksha Kireetam
c. Rudraksha wearing below waist (in yantra-Mantra-Tantra prayogas)

iv) Internal use of Rudraksha

For medical use of Rudraksha, honey coloured beads are the best, although they are available in white, black and mixed colours. Some of the preparations of Rudraksha which could be taken internally under observation of an Ayuvedic Doctor are–

(i) For tongue cracks, tastelessness and heaviness, gargling by Rudraksha's decoction has been found to be very effective.

(ii) Ten Rudraksha beads boiled with 200 ml. til oil and nine garlic pieces for 30 minutes and filtered. This filtered oil can be used by little warming up and applied on chest for cure of pneumonia and chest pains of spasmatic nature.

(iii) By keeping shanmukhi Rudraksha in a cup of boiling milk overnight a drink may be prepared and can be taken internally for 40 day for the treatment of mental weakness and also to improve the memory.

Latest Developments

Although the power of Rudraksha therapy has been known since ages of 5000 years, it is proved scientifically by the research done by a group of Scientists headed by Dr. Suhas Roy of Indian Institute of Technology, New Delhi in collaboration with Department of Biochemistry, Electrical engineering and Psychology of different Universities. They have proved that Rudraksha therapy has powerful electromagnetic, paramagnetic and inductive properties varying for different facets (Mukhi : The number of divisions on the surface) and on wearing particular facets of the Rudraksha beads, specific electrical impulses are sent to brain activating certain positive brain centres (brain chemical) thereby causing transformation in the personality, outlook, charisma and confidence of the wearer. They also proved that after wearing Rudraksha beads, the heart beat becomes normal, it smoothens the amount of blood going to the brain and with the help of these heads a kind of tranquility concentration and focus can be easily achieved which are elaborately discussed below:

Electrical Properties : The human body can be considered as a complex bio-electronic circuit consisting of the whole of "nervous system and all other organs residing inside the human body." Number of electrical impulses is generated by the human body due to different reflex actions taking place, continuous pumping of heart for blood circulation, neurons and nervous system etc. The ability to send out subtle electrical impulses & inductive vibrations and act as a Dielectric as in a capacitor to store electrical energy known as Bioelectricity. All the work of our sense organs depend on the subtle flow of Bioelectricity current. Thus all the actions our body performs are effectively controlled. The bioelectric current is produced due to the difference in the energy levels of different body parts. This smooth flow of bioelectric current causes the properly controlled functioning of the body parts.

Bio Electric Circuit : There is a third element in the body and brain called the Bio Electronic circuit Interface, that of the mind. Any activity that can produce stress or maladjustment can throw the streamlined activity, the Electronic circuit of the body & mind out of gear. Human beings and all living beings are prone to stress continuously in the continuous fight for survival and prosperity.

In modern age with intense competition the stress levels have increased tremendously. Almost every individual has problems of stress and its related ailments like insomnia, alcoholism, depression, maladjustments, heart diseases, skin diseases etc. Any Doctor will confirm that almost 95% of the ailments are Psychosomatic or stress related. When there is stress or maladjustment corresponding, stress signals are sent to the Central Nervous systems, there is an increased activity or abnormal of Neurons and Neuro transmitters. The magnitude of change will depend on the cause and specific case. When such a thing occurs and it occurs continuously, streamlined flow of electrical signals throughout the Mind-Body interface is disrupted and it makes us feel uncomfortable and we are not able to act with our full efficiency. Our blood circulation becomes non-ideal and we feel various illnesses. Unfortunately, this happens all the time.

Rudraksha beads act as a Stabilizing Anchor. Rudraksha beads' electrical property can be broadly categorized into:

Resistance : There is continuous and subtle flow of bioelectrical signal throughout the body due to potential difference between parts of the body. Rudraksha beads of particular Mukhis or Facets have a definitive factor of resistance. It is measured in Ohms. When these beads resist the flow of bioelectrical impulses a specific ampere of current flow is generated depending on the factor of resistance. This acts in tandem with heart beat, streamlining it and sending out specific impulses to brain. These impulses stimulate certain positive brain chemicals and make us feel better, more confidant, poised and more energetic. It has been observed that specific Mukhis or Facets of Rudraksha beads send out specific signals acting on a particular brain chemical and thereby effecting specific positive changes in personality.

Capacitance or the Dielectric Properties : Rudraksha beads act as dielectric (i.e.) as a storage of electrical energy. This property of Rudraksha makes it capable in stabilizing and anchoring the Bioelectric current. The values are measured in units of Farad. This property is very helpful in controlling hyperactivity, palpitations of heart, streamlining heartbeat etc. Due to stress when there is increased physical activity, heart beats faster and the overall activities of hormones and nervous system increase. This causes increase energy levels or increase in potential difference. As a result of this, the magnitude of the Bioelectric Current increases. Rudraksha beads acting as Dielectric store this excess Bioelectric Energy, thereby streamlining the overall activity to normalcy.

Inductance : Rudraksha beads by its permanent magnetic properties, observed to send out inductive vibrations with frequencies measured in units of Henry (Volt Seconds/ Ampere). This perhaps is the reason why people have felt better even when Rudraksha beads do not touch them physically.

Magnetic Properties : Rudraksha beads have both Paramagnetic and Diamagnetic with the most important property of Dynamic Polarity. We all are most probably aware of the beneficial healing properties of magnets. Magnetic healing is becoming extremely popular off late and everyone who have been using magnets for healing have been getting the benefits and found overall betterment and rejuvenation. Rudraksha beads retain most of the properties of Magnets but it is unparallel in one aspect, that of the ability to change its polarity or the property of Dynamic polarity. The basic way of healing is based on the fact that when the passage of arteries and veins which carry blood to and from heart to all the parts of the body is blocked or reduced due to variety of reasons, various illnesses creep. Blood carries oxygen and energy to various parts of the body and cleanses it off waste materials. Any disruption in the smooth flow of blood circulation is bound to cause illnesses.

We experience pain and uneasiness due to improper blood circulation. Every cell in the blood as well as the Arteries and veins are charged either positively or negatively. Magnets have the poles Positive (+) and Negative (-). When magnets are passed on various parts of the body the opposite poles of the magnets and that of cells get attracted and there is an expansion of the passage. The arteries and veins open up to facilitate streamlined blood circulation. When there is a streamlining of blood circulation most of the illnesses get automatically healed and we feel better and rejuvenated. But with magnets, the polarity is fixed. When magnets are brought near a particular part of the body it opens up only those sections of veins and arteries where there is a matching of polarities hence complete healing and streamlining of blood circulation cannot be ensured. We experience healing and feel better but we can still go much further with Dynamic Polarity of Rudraksha beads.

Dynamic Polarity : Rudraksha has the ability to-change its polarity. This in turn is by virtue of its property, Diamagnetism. Diamagnetism is termed as the ability of any material to acquire temporary Magnetic property in presence of an external magnetic field. The polarity of the charge induced is opposite to that of the external field inducing the charge. Blood circulation and heart beat automatically induce a magnetic field around the body and particularly the heart region. Bioelectricity automatically gives raise to Biomagnetism depending on the polarity of the induced magnetic field. Rudraksha bead acquires a polarity that is opposite to the inducing field. As a result of this, the opening up passages of arteries and veins are far better than that of magnets. Much better healing and rejuvenation are experienced.

The powerful anti ageing properties of Rudraksha beads have been mentioned in various literatures. This is mainly because of the Dynamic Polarity of the Rudraksha a bead thus the healing powers of Rudraksha are far superior to that of Magnets. In some sense, Rudraksha beads can be termed to have some additional life or intelligence as against magnet.

References

Anonymous, 1973, *The Alkaloids*, edited by R.H., Manske, Academic Press, London.

Armstrong, W.P., 1991, *Ornament*, 15:66-69.

Armstrong, W.P., 1998, *Botanical Jewelery*, Spring, New York, U.S.A.

Bhattacharya, S.K. Debnath, P.K. Pandey, V.B. and Sanyal, A.K., 1975, *Planta Medica*, Vol. 28:174-177.

Bhuyan, P., Khan, M.L. and Tri., R.S., 2002, *Current Science* Vol. 83, No. 11(1): 1-6.

Bose. T.K., Das, P. and Maiti, G.G., 1998, *Trees of the World*, Regional Plant Resource Centre, Bhubaneshwar, Orissa, Vol. I: 190.

Chatterjee Ashima and Pakrashi, S.C. 1994, *The treatise on Indian Medicinal Plants*, NISCARE, CSIR, New Delhi, Vol. 2.

Francis, Peter, Jr., 1984, *Economic Botany*, 38 (2): 194-204.

Khan, M.L., Upadhyaya, K., Singha, L.B., 2002, *Current Sicence*, 82:375-376.

Nadkarni, K.M., 1954, *Indian Meteria Medica*, Popular Book Depot, Bombay.

Pandey V.B., Bhattacharya, 1985, *Phytochemistry*, Vol. 14:2727-2728

Prajapati, N.D., Purohit, S.K. Sharma, A.K., Kumar, T.2003, *A Hand Book of Medicinal Plants: A complete source Book*, Agrobios, Jodhpur, Rajasthan.

Rao, R.R. and Haridasan, K., 1983, *An Assessment of the Tress of India*, edited by Jain, S.K. and Rao, R.R., BSI Howarah, West Bengal.

Sharma, P.V., 1983, *Dravyaguna Vijnana*, Chowkhamba Bharati Academcy, Varanasi.

Singh, R.K. and Gopinath, 1999, *Phyto-therapy Research*. Vol. 13 (5): 448-450.

Singh, R.K., Acharya, S.B. and Bhattacharya, S.K., 2000, *Phyto-therapy Research*, Vol. 14 (1): 36-39.

Swamy, K.S., 2000, Researches in *Ayurveda past and present*, Edited by VBL Gaur and S.K. Sharma, Jaipur Publication Scheme, Jaipur.

Chapter 9

Rudraksh – The Purest form of Cosmic Energy

❑ **Sunil Sobti**

Introduction

Rudraksh is formed by association of two words, 'RUDRA' and 'AKSHA'. Rudra is the name of Lord Shiva. Aksha means 'eye'. It is said that the plant of Rudraksh is originated from the tear drops from the eyes of Lord Shiva. As per the Vedic scriptures, Rudraksh can nullify the effects of malefic planets to a great extent. Shastras say: *Rudraksh of any mukhis can never do any harm to the wearer unlike Navratnas, which have to be carefully chosen.* No other necklace or bead is as auspicious and powerful as rudraksh. Rudraksh comes in different mukhis or the clefts or furrows on the surface. Shastras speak of 1 to 38 mukhis but normally 1 to 14 mukhis are used for astrological benefits. Each bead has a different effect on you, depending on the number of mukhis it has. Each rudraksh is individualistic and has to be carefully matched with one's horoscope for it to be beneficial.

Tantra, Yantra and Mantra with Rudraksh give much importance to Rudraksh. Vedas have given special weightage to Rudraksh, as it is believed that Rudraksh has originated from the tears of lord Shiva. Rudraksh has tremendous energy and power. Rudraksh is best known for its biomedical properties and in controlling stress, hypertension and blood pressure. Rudraksh is available mainly in Nepal and Malaysia. The chain of 108 beads or 50 beads if worn and worshipped, provides all types of benefits. Therefore, it is important that Rudraksh should always be respected and kept pure. One should not touch it with dirty hands and must be removed before entering the toilets. It is a blessing to mankind. It is believed that one who wears Rudraksh on their bodies, cannot be affected by sins. Even if, one wears Rudraksh on his body, without doing worship and chanting the sacred mantra, does not get near any sinful deed or thought.

Rudraksh is available in three categories

1. The biggest of rudraksh beads is 2.4 inches and is round. It is available in Java, Sumatra and China.
2. Rudraksh of middle category ranges from 1.75 inches. These are available in the heads that come 32 Mukhas.
3. They are the smallest and their size is less than 1.50 inches. In this category, the bead comes in the size of black pepper. These are the costliest of all.

How to identify the real Rudraksh?

1. If you place a real rudraksh bead in a full glass of water, it would drown in water.
2. Boil the rudraksh in water for continuous 6 hours. If it is real rudraksh there would be rudraksh bead, else if it is artificial or two rudrakshas are joined together they will get separated.
3. Rudraksh should not be confused with the shape and size. One should carefully examine whether the beads are well defined, *corns and contours are natural*, there are no cracks near the bead has a good health. Smaller size is also considered to be very auspicious.
4. Rudraksh bead shall not be broken from any end.

Rudraksh is of special importance in religious ceremonies and prayers of God – Goddess gets one faced and 9 to 14 faced Rudraksh. One faced rudraksh is very rare and Rudraksh chain (mala) is therefore, considered ideal for pooja purposes. A chain of 50 beads is placed over the heart, while the chain of 16 beads should be worn on the forehead.

Rudraksh should surely be placed in one's place of worship at home. This rosary is effective that you can yourself experience it. When a Sadhak places such articles and uses them then a time comes when he realizes their power.

While stringing the beads, each bead is energized with Shiva Mantra and then it should be kept in pure water chanting the Sadyojaat Mantra which is as follows.

"Om Sadyojaatam Prapadyaami Sadyojaatave Namo Namaha"

Benefits of Rudraksh

The Rudrakshs are worn for their specific benefits. These are much more powerful and can help achieve wonders, if *energized and empowered* the right way. Rudraksh of different mukhis pleases the corresponding planets. It may be sufficient to go in for only for those mukhis whose ruling planets, cause malefic effects.

It has been proved that wearing Rudraksh regulates heartbeat and gives positive effect, maintaining blood pressure, removes stress, anxiety, depression. It is also proved that Rudraksh has anti-ageing property as well as different mukhi's from 1 mukhi to 15 mukhi beads have specific powers and have powerful Electromagnetic, Paramagnetic and Inductive properties that vary for different mukhi or facets. Every human being & other living things have their own Aura, a field of energy that surrounds people & other living things, reflects the energy of the spirit in that body, this energy extends about *two to four inches* around the body & a light or pastel shade. It contains every colour & shade in the rainbow & usually extends 2-5 inches from the body. Its colours, textures & patterns reveal much information about emotional, mental, physical, spiritual, karmic, environmental & relational states. As Aura is like a *thumbprint*; it is completely individual & expresses who you really are in your entire splendor. When Rudraksh beads are worn, they interface and integrate with the human body at a silent subtle level of consciousness. Due to their Dielectric and Magnetic properties, the Rudraksh beads initiate and effect positive change in the Bio-electrical system of the human body in a life-supporting manner. As a result of this change in electrical makeup of our body, positive change is also initiated in our bio-chemical System.

There are no compulsions to wear a specific bead of rudraksh as one can wear the combination of all beads and one can also wear a pendant of any specific facet of beads or a mix of different facet of beads as it does not have any negative effects unlike gemstones, which can cause a greater level of harm. The human body is basically a bio-electronic circuit, blood circulation; the transmission of various impulses and the continuous movement of neurons and neurotransmitters in the brain generates electrical impulses which collectively make bio-electricity. It is believed and proved that rudraksh beads have certain electro-magnetic and inductive properties and when worn over the heart they send out corresponding signals differing for different mukhis to the brain, activating or controlling certain brain chemicals and neurotransmitters thereby inducing states of mind as described in ancient scriptures. For example, the mental agitation and Dopamine levels. Increased amount of dopamine cause over activity of neurons resulting in mental agitation, restlessness, tension, fear, lack of control etc.; conversely decreased levels 'of dopamine, result in peace, tranquility, stability etc. Of those who wore 5 mukhi rudraksh the low levels of Serotonin was seen in their blood. One such neurotransmitter causes depression, worry, lack of energy, low self-esteem and raised high which gave them energy, drive, high levels of confidence and self esteem etc. Of those who wore 1 mukhi and 12 mukhi Rudraksh were also found to be higher in Serotonin level.

The activity of neurons in the right part of the brain was found to be high in the wearer of 14 mukhi rudraksh bead (right part of the brain controls abstract and lateral thinking as against logical and structural thinking of left part of brain). This perhaps is the reason behind the change in personality and attitudes of the wearer of different types of rudraksh beads. When the persons get a positive, confident frame of mind the impact goes deep into his subconscious mind sending out powerful, positive vibrations thereby changing the way nature and others react to him/her.

Rudraksh beads act as a stabilizing newscaster, which can control the bio-electronic circuit of our body. Rudraksh beads also have Paramagnetic and Diamagnetic properties with the most important property of Dynamic polarity. Rudraksh beads have the properties of magnets but it is unparallel in one aspect, that of the ability to change it's polarity or the property of Dynamic Polarity. Medically, it has been proved that rudraksh has very powerful anti-ageing properties because of the Dynamic Polarity of the Rudraksh bead thus, the healing powers of rudraksh are far superior to that of magnets. In some sense, rudraksh beads can be termed to have some additional life or intelligence as against magnets.

●

Chapter 10

Rudraksh: An Overview of Medicinal & Spiritual Significance

❑ **Tanay Setha & Kapil Khanna**

Why should one wear Rudraksh in today's context?

Rudraksh bead, meaning "eye of Shiva" in Sanskrit, is a seed of fruit from the rudraksha tree (*Elaeocarpus ganitrus*) growing in the wild in Nepal, South of Himalayas, Indonesia and scantily in Varanasi, Dehradun and Haridwar.

The beads have different faces (mukhi) from 1 to 14 which are dividing lines from mouth to tail end of the bead. Faces higher than 14 upto 23 have been spotted but do not find mention in holy scriptures like *Shiva Purana, Padma Purana, Devi Bhagwad, Rudrakshajabalopanishad* etc. Similarly, Gauri Shankar (Two rudraksha beads joined together), Trijuti (3 beads joined together), Ganesh Gauri, Ganesh Sawar etc., do not feature in these epics but have become commonly acceptable as divinely blessed due to their properties and experiences of people. One mukhi round bead is nearly impossible.to get therefore all stories about it (including that Late Mrs. Indira Gandhi used to wear 1 mukhi mala) are not entirely true. People are generally more anxious about rare things and this author has several interesting observations from across the world and would like to mention them in summary form. Forget about 1 mukhi round rudraksha, if it exists, only Lord Shiva has the right over it. However, a substitute form of 1 mukhi half moon shape from Rameshwaram has now been accepted by all. Some of the reputed ashrams too selling this round 1 mukhi only show ignorance of the seller and the buyer.

Rudraksha unlike other forms of healing objects give effect only if sanctified using beeja mantras or panchakshar mantra "Namah Shivaya". Unless blessed by the respective God which the rudraksha represents, it would not give full effects except the biomedical effects. Therefore, the spiritual level of rudraksha should never be undermined.

Rudraksha is a healing bead with divine characteristics proven over several thousand years of our culture. From Lord Shiva Himself all spiritual and great personalities have adorned themselves with rudraksha and with the benefits that people of modern age have derived from these, Rudra Centre has hundreds of testimonials from all over the world. It is beyond any doubt that this powerful bead has the potential to become a powerful tool to overcome stress and to combat fear.

As regards to the scientific or intellectual explanations other than related to faith or traditional wisdom, the following explanations should be considered as basic parameters for the use of rudraksha.

It brings us close to the Nature. 'Rudraksha' is the seed of a fruit from the rudraksha tree. Trees represent nature hence, if the seed closely touches our body, we become one with nature, just like all others in the animal kingdom.

Feeling of Universal being is created. Rudraksha mala is also called *Aksha mala. All letters (akshars) of Sanskrit language are based on sounds and we all know that Lord Shiva's musical instrument Damaru created the Pratyahars and from these 50 letters were generated. The Akshar name given to letters denotes those letters. Akshar, like sounds, cannot be destroyed.* The rudraksha seeds in a mala (also called Aksha mala) represent these sounds and a feeling of belongingness to cosmos is perceived by wearing it and a person wearing rudraksha represents a part of cosmos.

Acupressure

Good for the heart. Constant stimulation of heart muscles by beads having smooth yet protruded surface keeps the blood pressure under control and hence it is considered good for the heart.

Watchful eye of Lord Shiva

Rudra-Aksha means eye of Shiva. If one wears rudraksha he/she is under protection of watchful eyes of Lord Shiva.

Biomedical benefits

The bio-medical and electro-magnetic properties of rudraksha are well known and scientifically proven and will give benefits to the body by improving their functions and keeping the diseases at bay. Like neem, tulsi, haldi and other herbal products, rudraksha is being evaluated world-wide by leading research laboratories and we should preserve our cultural heritage by accepting the traditional beliefs.

Blessings of different Gods

Different mukhi rudraksha have their respective Gods as Pradhan Devatas from Lord Surya, Hanuman, Vishnu, Brahma, Durga and Kartikeya and of course, Lord Shiva himself and by wearing them we get blessings of all of them.

Planetary blessings

Each rudraksha (one to nine mukhi) has its own ruling planet. Ten mukhi and 11 mukhi are beyond any planetary configuration. Hindu astronomers consider 14 galactical cosmos (14 Bhuwans) and therefore, rudraksha has the blessings of Planetary Gods.

Confession of one's sins and for fearless life

If a human being wants to restart his life after committing a sin, where does he/she go. All of our epics on rudraksha describe the potentiality of each mukhi rudraksha acting as divine objects before which we can confess our sin and restart a fresh life free of regrets and remorse. Probably that is the reason why rudraksha are considered to be relievers of stress and strain of life.

Spiritual Significance

Compared to any other mala, a rudraksha mala for japa and sadhana is most auspicious. For enhancing spirituality and attaining Riddhi and Siddhi at all levels, rudraksha is the most effective medium.

Rudraksha is an Upa-Guru

If you have not found a guru so far or even if you have a Guru, rudraksha will act like your Upa-Guru or a teacher substitute to show you the path and enlighten you to reach higher levels of wisdom and karma.

Various physical & mental problems

The ancient rudraksha beads are now gaining importance in the present era as their healing properties are being identified and recommended by Rudraksha Therapists for various physical and mental problems. Rudraksha beads (botanical name : *Eleaocarpus ganitrus*) are the dried fruits of the rudraksha tree found mainly in Java and Sumatra, Assam, Himalayan region, Sikkim, Nepal and Bhutan. Talking to this, Pune-based Dr. Madhuri Mahadevan, a clairvoyant and a Feng Shui Consultant as well as a Rudraksha Therapist says, "For thousands of years the merits and powers of the rudraksha beads have been documented and detailed in the holy Puranas and Upanishads."

According to Dr. Madhavan, wearing the sacred rudraksha beads brings one to the alpha state of present moment living. Dr. Madhuri points out, "The ancient discipline of rudraksha recommendation is as simple as it is complicated". She further states that today, there are many rudraksha therapy facilities in India that recommend rudraksha beads by combining ancient Vedic Knowledge with modern scientific proof and confirmed experiences, continually proving the effectiveness of wearing rudraksh beads.

Stressing on the scientific aspect of the beads, she firmly believes modern science has shown that the *electromagnetic nature of rudraksha beads affect our neurophysiology in a specific manner that allows control of heart beat, blood pressure, stress levels, hypertension and at the same time relieves anxiety, depression and neurotic conditions.*

Anti-aging properties have also been discovered, based on the natural electromagnetism of rudraksha beads. She calls rudraksha Nature's gift to mankind and a panacea for all illnesses falling into the category of using herbs and plants for counteracting not only the evil effects of planets but all at clinical level for illnesses such as hypertension, cancer and AIDS, and many others.

As a Rudraksh Therapist and a clairvoyant, Dr. Madhavan also suggested the usage of rudraksha beads to several clients suffering from cancer and AIDS. "I recommend the usage of rudraksha beads externally by wearing them, and internally by drinking milk to which rudraksh beads have been added and boiled." She adds that these beads help tremendously as *supportive therapy* and nullifies all side effects of medication as well as speed up their efficacy. Wearing them also gives strength to the patient to cope with the medication.

However, Dr. Madhavan stresses on the need for further scientific research and analysis in order to understand their benefits in the field of health and medicine, for the good of all mankind.

Rudraksh : A Therapeutic Approach

Large genus (Elaeocarpus. Linn.) of trees belonging to the family Eleocarpaceae, distributed from South and East Asia through Malaysia to Australia and Pacific Islands. About 25 species occur in India. This medium sized tree also grows in Nepal, Bihar, Bengal, Assam, Madhya Pradesh and Maharashtra. But the author has noticed its presence in the Nicobars, especially in Great Nicobar Island. Morphologically, its leaves are oblong-lanceolate, subentire, nearly glabrous. Flowers are white in dense recemes, arising mostly from old leaf aisles. Drupe, deep or bluish-purple, globose or obovoid (0.5 – 1.0 inch diameter) enclosing a hard, longitudinally grooved, tubercled normally five-celled stone in which five seeds are embedded.

The stones are cleaned and polished, sometimes stained and used as beads for rosaries, bracelets and other ornamental objects. They are frequently set in gold and stones with fewer or more than five cells, fetch high prices. Rudraksha beads have mukhis or 'faces' that differ in number and this is what distinguishes them from each other. Almost all beads are five-faced, with a very small percentage being more or less.

The therapeutic and spiritual attributes of a rudraksha bead is dependent on the number of 'faces' it exhibits. Beads which have a single face to about twenty-one faces have been found. Rudraksha are treasured by the followers of the God of the Hindu trinity, Shiva, the destroyer. According to the

Shiva Purana, it is impossible to describe adequately, the benefits of wearing rudraksha even in 100 years.

In Ayurveda, Rudraksha is useful in the treatment of high blood pressure, allergies, neurological diseases, asthma, diabetes, cancer and many other Raktavaha Srotadhikara (blood circulatory disorders) and Manas Rogas (mental disorders), due to its Guru (heaviness), Snigdha Guna (greasy nature) Mahura Rasa, Madhura Vapaka and Sita Virya (cooling properties) and Vata Pitta samaka pharmacodynamic action. On the basis of these pharmacodynamic properties and actions, the significance of various types of beads of rudraksha (actually a phalasthi (fruit) which is the used part of this tree) can be considered as follows:

External use

External therapeutic uses of rudraksha can be performed by Darsana (by gazing on, like tratak in yoga) and by Sparsana (by wearing, and pressing the beads).

The application of lepa of Pancha Mukhi beads leads to pacification of Pitta or Dahasamana, just as chandana is, and applied on Masurika eruption.

- Wearing of Eka Mukhi (one faced) beads fulfils desire.
- Wearing of Dwi Mukhi (two faced) ensures control of desires.
- Rubbing of Tri Mukhi (three faced) in milk and applied to the eye helps eye ailments.
- Wearing of Chatur Mukhi (four faced) can increase grasping power and intelligence.
- Wearing of Pancha Mukhi (five faced) increases mental peace, normalizes blood circulation. This type is also used as an ornament.
- Wearing of Shasta Mukhi (six faced) beads increases memory retention.
- Wearing of Sapta Mukhi (seven faced) increases will power.
- Wearing of Ashta Mukhi (eight faced) beads increases concentration, develops knowledge and removes obstacles in proposed plans and works.
- Wearing of Dasa Mukhi (ten faced) is useful in spiritual enlightenment and reduces mental stress and strain.

Rudraksha is also known as Bhuta Nashana (literally, destroying ghosts) due to its action in relieving mental disorders. Wearing rudraksha benefits in various ways, depending on the number of faces. On the basis of pharmacological experiments by experts, it has been proven that rudraksha is beneficial in the treatment of neurological and mental disorders. It has been found that, smaller or medium-sized rudraksha are most effective for wearing and japam. Moreover, while performing japam (meditation with chanting), applying a little pressure on the beads with the thumb and middle finger improves blood circulation in the eye and brain (acupressure theory). Rudraksha beads can be worn on the wrist, forearms, neck, chest, head, forehead, earlobes and around the midriff. A rudraksha mala can be made of 108, 54, 36, 27 or 18 beads. Only strong, well-formed and grooved rudraksha beads should be used. One natural hole through the centre is the best.

Form of Uses

The rudraksha beads are taken orally and externally in the form of Him (frozen), Kvatham, Milk, Bhasma (ash), Vibhuti, Tailam (oil), Kalkam, Mandap, Kirtanan, mala etc.

Internal use

Rudraksha is also administered in powdered form in dosage of 3-5 gm or mixed with other Ayurvedic herbs. Internal intake improves their effectiveness and shortens the treatment period. The systemic action of rudraksha is as follows:

It acts as an anti-convulsant and analgesic on the nervous system.

- **Three** faced beads are useful in curing indigestion. Both three faced and five faced beads are effective in the treatment of circulatory system disorders like hypertension. They affect the respiratory system by acting as a bronchodilator and are useful in the treatment of dyspnoea. They are effective in the treatment of asthma and in treating malaria.
- **Four** faced rudraksha beads are effective in treating skin disorders.
- **Six** faced beads are particularly effective in the treatment of epilepsy and hysteria.
- **Nine** faced beads are effective in the treatment of urino-genital disorders, and aid in the prevention of

miscarriages. Moreover, these beads are also useful in lowering the body temperature and act as an antipyretic agent during fever.

- **Ten** faced beads are used in reducing mental stress and strain. They are hepatotonic for Liver in the gastrointestinal system and are useful in the treatment of jaundice and other hepatic disorders. Ten-faced beads also control whooping cough and are effective in treating temperature regulation related disorders.

Precautions

To maintain their potency, rudraksha beads must be kept off the ground and wrapped in either wool or silk when not in use. Cleaning the beads with sandal wood oil once a month is also recommended.

1. The bigger beads are the best for both medicinal purposes and worshipping whereas smaller sized rudraksha are more potent for wearing and performing japam.
2. Only strong, well-formed and grooved rudrakshas are recommended. The ones with a natural hole through the centre are the most effective.
3. It is found that rudraksha must be used for more than 40 days, to achieve the desired results.

Before using rudraksha, one must test its genuineness by the following:

- The central hole of the rudraksha should be natural.
- When an original rudraksha is kept between two clean copper coins, it will move slightly due to the magnetic effect.
- When a rudraksha is kept in water, a little heat is discharged after a few hours and the colour of water changes.
- Genuine Rudraksha sinks when put in water.
- Only a genuine rudraksha must be selected, as it has great medicinal and spiritual attributes.

Rudraksh is recommended for physical and mental ailments. To verify this recommendation in scientific explanation, it is felt by the author to research on evaluation of rudraksha.

References

The wealth of India, Raw Materials, Vol. III, D.E. CSIR New Delhi 1952,

Dictionary of Economic Products, DEP – III, 205, Commercial Products (CP) 511, Hooker's Flora of British India (F1, Br. Ind.) I, 400,

Kirt & Basu I, 404 Shruit Sharma in Indian Express, S.K. Bhattacharya et al. Pharmacological investigations on *Elaeocarpus ganitrus*,

Plant Media, October 1985 Dravya Guna Vigyan by Priyavrat Sharma Chaukhambha Bharti Academy, 1983,

Dr. Raakhee Mehra, M.D. (Ay.), Ph.D., Officer in_charge, Tribal Health Care Research Project (Ay.),

Car Nicobar, A & N Islands, India.

The Saiva Upanishads

Rudra of the Upanishads

Some people think that Rudra is a malevolent, terrific deity who causes destruction. They believe that Rudra is a God of punishment. It is not so. Rudra is the God who bestows prosperity and destroys suffering. He is a benevolent Deity who confers auspiciousness, offspring and cattle. He is the bringer or source of prosperity.

Shiva or Rudra means He who removes sin or suffering. The names Bhava, Sarva, Pasupati, Urga, Mahadeva, Isana and Asani are applied to Rudra. Pasupati means the Lord or Protector of cattle.

In the Vedas, you will find prayers such as, "O Rudra! May we increase in offspring." "Thou, O Rudra, art the most eminent of beings, the strongest of the strong wielder of the thunder-bolt; protect us, carry us happily across our calamity, drive away all evils." "Remove us from whatever sins we have done." Therefore, Rudra is not a terror-inspiring God, but bestows welfare or prosperity. He is the one great Lord of the Universe.

Rudra is the ideal of medicants, because Rudra alone, of all the deities, is spoken of in the scriptures as the medicant God. He is mentioned as having the ascetic water pot in the Rig Veda hymns.

You will find in the Svetasvatara Upanishad, Chapter III "There is one Rudra only who rules all the worlds by His powers. There is no one besides Him who can make Him the second. He is present inside the hearts of all beings. He creates the entire world and finally withdraws them into Himself."

Rudra represents here Para Brahma or the Supreme Self, the Infinite or the Absolute.

Rudra after having created all objects, draws together or takes them all back into Himself at the end of time, i.e., during cosmic Pralaya or dissolution.

Rudra is the destructive aspect of Shiva. There are eleven rudras in the cosmic hierarchy. Esoterically, the pranas (the ten senses) and the mind represent the eleven Rudras. Sri Hanuman is a manifestation or aspect of Rudra only.

In Shiva Purana, Rudra is another name for Shiva. Rudra is one who destroys the sins and removes the miseries of His devotees and confers on them wisdom and bliss. Rudra is the Antaryamin or indweller of all beings. He witnesses silently the actions and thoughts of men and dispenses the fruits of their actions.

"O, Rudra with Thy form which is auspicious, which is not dreadful and which manifests what is holy, with that all blessed form, appear to us, O Dweller among the mountains."

The Rudraksajabalopanisad

This. Upanishad which is the 88th among the 108 Upanishads and forms part of the Samaveda takes the form of a discourse between Bhusunda and Kalagnirudra regarding the part played by rudraksa in the attainment of the state of the Brahman. Although Bhusunda was himself an accomplished Yogin of the high order who had discharged all his duties and had nothing more to do in this world for the attainment of Kaivalya of the incorporeal type, still, for the regeneration of the deluded and the ignorant, he approached Lord Kalagnirudra with a prayer for the exposition of the rules prescribed for the wearing of rudraksha beads and the fruit attainable so as to enable seekers to attain the right kind of knowledge , with a mind thoroughly purified through sincere devotion to him as such knowledge is the sine qua non for the attainment of the state of the Paramatman, Rudra, the main support of the phenomenal world, preparatory to the attainment of the state of the formless and the supportless non differentiated Brahman.

Thereupon Bhusunda asked the reputed Kalagnirudra : What, pray, is the genesis of the rudraksa? What is the fruit attainable through the wearing of the same?

Lord Kalagnirudra replied unto him: For bringing about the destruction of the Tripura I had to close my eyes. Thereupon drops of tears fell on the earth from my eyes. Those drops became Rudrakshas. For the sake of the regeneration of all beings, I have ordained that, by the mere uttering the name of various types of rudraksh, peace & salvation is gifted by me to a person.

Fruit of wearing rudraksha and the uttering of prayer with it: By being worn by the devotee of Rudra, it will remove all sins committed by day and night. By looking at it religious merit will be attained a hundred thousand fold, and by wearing it ten thousand fold. By wearing it, a man will attain a hundred crores of units of religious merit. By uttering prayers as Japa with its help and by wearing the rudraksha a man will attain religious merit to the tune of a lakh of crores of thousands and a lakh of crores of hundreds respectively.

- Sri Mad Devi Bhaghvatam

Chapter VI

If anybody holds rudraksham on his head, he gets koti times the fruit; on his ears, ten koti times fruit; on his neck, one hundred kofitirues the fruit; on his holy thread, ayta times the fruit; on his arm, one lakh koti times the fruit and if one wears rudraksham on one's wrist, one attains moksha. Whatever acts, mentioned in the Vedas be performed with Rudraksham on, the fruits obtained are unbounded.

If anybody holds rudraksham together with pearls, Prabala, crystal, silver, gold and gem (*lapis lazuli*), he becomes a manifestation of Shiva. If a body, through laziness even, holds rudraksham, the sin cannot touch him as darkness cannot come near light. If anybody makes japam of a mantra with a rudraksha rosary, he gets unbounded results. Such a merit giving rudraksha, if one such rudraksham be not found on anyone's body, his life becomes useless, like a man who is void of tripundrak (three curved horizontal marks made on the forehead by the worshippers of Shiva). If one simply washes his head all over with rudraksham on, he gets the fruit of bathing in the Ganges. There is no doubt in this. One-faced rudraksham, the five-faced, eleven-faced and fourteen-faced rudrakshams are highly meritorious and entitled to worship by all. The rudraksham is sankara made manifest; so it is always worshipped with devotion. The greatness of rudraksham is such as it can make a king out of a poor man.

Srimaddevibhagavat 11th Skand Chapter IV

God said–

19 – 20 Those men who wear either the rosary of rudraksha or even one bead on their head, get rid of all pains, sorrows and sins and attain all the credits and fabulous money. Such men on chanting the names of Shiva become superior to all other men.

22 Wearer of rudraksha on hair tuft of the crown, in ear, in neck, in hand and in abdomen attains the status of Shiva, Visnu and Brahma.

23 All the deities, saints, etc. reside in the rudraksha if worn with devotion.

24 Saints, religious persons and all the pious souls born in the genealogy of such persons feel pleasure and become pious.

25 – 26 According to Jabala instinct for wearing Rudraksha results only after attaining the perfection of Vedas and blessings of Lord Shiva during preceding births.

27 O son, the benefits and greatness of rudraksha beads famous in all the three worlds are studied by all the saints and by me.

28 – 29 Rudraksha-wearing provides hundred million times more punya (merits) than that accrues on touching and seeing it. If a man does chanting (japa) on it, he attains several trillion times benefits. It is an eternal truth and therefore, it is needless to speak any more on its benefits.

14 – 16 The berry (of the rudraksha) should touch the middle finger. Then in the proper order one should mutter, moving one's hand, and again and again touching the central bead of the rosary.

One should count the number of the mantras (sacred word/name/formula) that are muttered. If they are not counted they are fruitless. One should mutter the names of all gods with (i.e. by counting the beads of) ones own rosary.

17 – 21 (If he after) being pure (mutters the mantras) in all sacred places the merit would be a crore-fold. He would obtain endless fruit if he mutters a mantra in honour of the image of Vishnu or Shiva or Ganapati or the Sun, on a pure ground, or at the pure root of a tree, in a cowpen, or in a house at a crossway.

The Lord Spoke

91 – O Kartikeya, hear correctly about the assignment and wearing of rudrakshas of different numbers of mouths. The merits (already) told are without the recital of a sacred hymn. The merits and the importance of the man who on the earth wears it to the accompaniment of a sacred hymn cannot be told.

92 – Now the sacred hymns are indicated:

Om Rudra ekavaktrasya
Om Kham dvivaktrasya
Om Ambum trivaktrasya
Om Hrim caturvaktrasya
Om Hram pancavaktrasya
Om Hrum sadvaktrsya
Om Hrah saptavaktrasya
Om Kam astavaktrasya
Om Jum navavaktrasya
Om Aksam dasavaktrasya
Om Srim ekadasavaktrasya
Om Hrim dvadasavaktrasya
Om Ksom trayodasavaktrasya
Om Nram chaturdasavaktrasya

Thus, the sacred hymns should be assigned in due order. A man who wears a rosary (of Rudrakshas) on his head or chest, walks, obtains at every step the fruit (of performance) of a horse sacrifice not otherwise.

93 - 99 – Man becomes equal to me by wearing Rudraksha of all mouths (i.e. by wearing Rudraksha having any number of mouths. Therefore, O son, with all efforts wear a rudraksha.

Chapter 11

Rudraksh for Health and Self Empowerment

❑ **M.S. Neeta & Dharam Deva Arya**

The tears of Lord Shiva that are Rudraksh, are the original Vedic beads of Power worn by the Yogis of India and the Himalayas for thousands of years to maintain health and to gain self-empowerment and fearless life on their path to enlightenment and liberation.

The Electromagnetic properties of the Rudraksh beads improve concentration, focus and mental stamina. Due to these properties, it was found that wearing Rudraksh beads around the heart reduced and controlled stress levels, blood pressure and hypertension resulting in the feeling of tranquility and calmness. Rudraksh beads were found to be ideal for focused meditation and other spiritual practices.

Historically, the positive effects that have been exhibited in the wearers neurophysiology, personality and physical health have resulted in their being used widely in the Eastern cultures of India, China and Japan by Hindus, Buddhists and followers of Zen.

It is remarkable to consider that natural beads of vegetable matter from the Rudraksh tree affect the human neurophysiology as described in the Vedic literature. However, recent scientific research has again found Vedic knowledge to be correct.

Though the powers of Rudraksh have been known as a phenomenon for thousands of years in Vedic knowledge, it is only since the late 1980s that they have become more prominent particularly after the research done by a group of scientists led by Dr. Subas Rai Ph.D. of the Institute of Technology University of Banaras, India.

A combined study to research the Biomedical implications of Rudraksh was conducted with the Departments of Biochemistry, Electrical Engineering, Psychiatry, General Medicine and Psychology. This study proved and documented the powers and effects of Rudraksh beads scientifically with reproducible results.

Research has proved that Rudraksh have powerful electromagnetic, paramagnetic and inductive properties that vary from the different mukhis or facets (the different number of divisions found on the surface of each bead). They also found that wearing or performing Japa with a particular mukhi or set of mukhis of the Rudraksh beads created specific electrical impulses that are sent to the brain through the process of galvanic skin response stimulating certain brain centres that transfer information.

This bioelectric stimulation affects the biochemical system in the brain creating a positive impact on the activity of neurotransmitters, dopamine and serotonin levels that is evidenced by the positive transformation in the personality, mindset, outlook, charisma and the confidence of the wearer.

It was also found that those wearing Rudraksh beads were able to experience reduced stress reaction to unexpected levels that were normally possible only with continued doses of tranquilizers.

In scientific terms, the Rudraksh beads are dielectric as they store electrical energy and they have permanent magnetic properties that change with the different mukhi beads. The complete list of all the properties found inherent in the Rudraksh beads include electromagnetism, para magnetism, diamagnetism and dynamic polarity or the ability to change polarity.

When Rudraksh beads are worn over the heart and Rudraksh Malas are revolved in Japa they interface and integrate with the human body at a silent subtle level of consciousness. Due to their dielectric and magnetic properties, the Rudraksh beads initiate and effect positive changes in our neurophysiology.

The Rudraksh effect brings the wearer into the alpha state of mental energy vibrations which is essential to gain self-empowerment, fearless life, enlightenment and liberation. (moksha)

The alpha state produced in the brain boosts the confidence and inner strength of the wearer significantly and as a result the heart beat, circulation, function of endocrine glands and activity of neurons and respiration is normalized in the physical body.

Supporting scientific evidence for these statements are again found in the published research papers by Subas Rai describing the beneficial powers of Rudraksh by virtue of electrical and magnetic properties that affect our central nervous system, automatic sympathetic and parasympathetic nervous systems and other organ systems in totality to maintain holistic health.

It was proven that wearing of Rudraksh controlled heart beat and had a positive effect on blood pressure, stress, anxiety, depression, palpitations and lack of concentration. It was also found that Rudraksh have anti-ageing properties based on their electromagnetism – which maintain the bioelectric potentials of the wearer.

Generations who have worn authentic Rudraksh beads have repeatedly confirmed that they have experienced considerable relief from the debilitating effects of high blood pressure, stress, hypertension, depression and other mind related problems including neurotic conditions.

In the evolution of spiritual consciousness, the holy Rudraksh beads are related to Absolute Field of Consciousness. They manifest in the relative field as an eternal triggering mechanism to be recognized by mankind and the womankind as and when we are awakened to higher states of consciousness in each lifetime.

The Srimaddevibhagavat 11th Skand Chapter V parts 25 and 26 states.

According to Jabala instinct for wearing Rudraksh results only after attaining the perfection of Vedas and blessings of Lord Shiva during preceding births.

Interpretation of this knowledge reflects the existence of memory of Rudraksh in our spiritual evolution from past lifetimes that can be triggered in a present lifetime.

In our experience, we have seen the initial Rudraksh effect triggered by the mere reading of the word Rudraksh in print or the physical sight or touch of a Rudraksh bead.

We have found this triggered memory affects men, women and children and runs throughout many populations in the world. From 4 years of age in India to people in their 50s and older in the United States and Europe such exponential observations have been reported. When the Rudraksh is recognized by those who are wakening upto higher states of consciousness and remembering on higher levels there is an unexplained need experienced to have Rudraksh in their lives again.

The Vedic Puranas also show that there are more powerful Rudraksh beads from 1 mukhi to 21 mukhi each capable of aligning our mind and the positive energies around us to specific aspects of health, happiness, spiritual fulfilment, prosperity, creativity, intuitive ability, material fulfilment, family harmony, attraction, self empowerment and fearless life.

The Srimaddevibhagavat gives us the needed explanation from Vedic knowledge regarding the unexplained attraction to Rudraksha beads. Modern day science shows us how the Rudraksha effect can help all the mankind function and perform better leading to a happy, healthy and more successful life.

●

Section V
BIBLIOGRAPHY

Chapter 12

Selected References Related to Studies on Rudraksh in India and Abroad

1. Acharya R.S. (1976) Shiva Puran. Sanskrit Institute, Bareily, Vol. I.p. 170
2. Bansal Abha (2004) Mysteries of Rudraksh. AIFS journal of Astrology (April-June 2004) p. 28.
3. Bhattacharya S.K, (1975) Pharmacological P.K. Debnath, V.B. Pandey Investigations on & S.K. Sanyal E. ganitrus, planta Medica. p. 175
4. Chand Lal (1975) Photochemistry Vol. 14 (2727).
5. Dhanvantri (1968) Ayurvedic Journal Bala Rognak.
6. Dhar M.L., Dhar M.M. (1968), B.N. Mehrotra & C. Roy Screening of Indian Medicinal Plants for Biological activity Part-I, Ind. J. Exptl. Biology. Vol. VI.p.232
7. Gupta S.P. (1983) MD Thesis (General Medicine) Study of Effect of Rudraksh (E. ganitrus) in Hypertension MD. Thesis (1983) IMS - Banaras Hindu University, Varanasi (U.P.)
8. Koul Maharaj Krishen (2001) Ruddy & Revered Rudraksh. Daily Excelsior (Sunday Magazine, 4th November) p.4
9. Kirtikar & Basu (1954) Indian Medical Plants. Vol. I.p.404
10. Lee David W (1991) Ultra Structural basis & Functions of iridescent blue colour of fruits in *Elaeocarpus*. *Nature* 349 : 260-262.
11. Lee David W (1997) Iridescent Blue Plants. American Scientist (Jan - Feb 1997).
12. Lee David W (1998) The Biology of Rudraksh. *Current Science* (Bangalore). Vol. 75(1): July 1998 : pp.26-30.

13. Lakhotia Ravinder (1998) Rattan, Rudraksh Aur Aap (in Hindi) Radha Pocket Books, Meerut (U.P.).
14. Nadkarni (1954) Indian Materia Medica p.473
15. Pandey V.B. & S.K. Bhattacharya (1985) Scientific Appraisal of Rudraksh : Chemical & Pharmacological Studies: Journal Research, Education Indian, Medicine. (Jan-June 1985).p.48
16. Rai Subas (2004) Rudraks: Properties & Biomedical Implications. Ganga-Kaveri Publishing Varanasi (UP) p. 197.
17. R. Venugopalan (2005) Rudraksha B. Jain Publication, New Delhi.
18. Rakesh (1998) Rudraksh Aur Rattan Mala (in Hindi) Sadhna Pocket Books, Delhi.
19. Raja Radhakant Deva (1987) Shabdhakalpdruma. Vol. 4. Naga Prakashan, New Delhi.
20. Sarkar P.K. (1972a) Effect of E. ganitrus Roxb Seeds on Blood Pressure. Indian Journal of Pharmacy Vol. IV : p. 128
21. Sarkar P.K. & Gupta S.S. (1972b) Studies with Ethyle acetate extract of E. ganitrus Roxb on Mammalian heart: Intact & Isolated preparations. Indian journal of Pharmacy Vol. IV.p.129
22. Sarkar P.K., Gupta S.S. & Bhattacharya S.S. (1973) Furturc Observations with E. ganitrus on normal & hypodermic heart. Indian journal of Pharmacy. Vol.IV.p.252
23. Sharma B.D. & M. Sanjappa (Editors) (1973) Flora of India Vol. 3 Botanical Survey of India; Kolkata.
24. Sharma B.D. (2005) Miracles of Rudraksh Therapy Mystic India Magazine, Vol. 6(6) pp. 44-46.
25. Sharma, B.D. (2008) Rudraksh Therapy: Rediscovered for Practice and Research (in Press).
26. Shubhakaran, K.T. (2000) Shri Rudram-Decoded: Mysteries of Vedas Revealed – Mantras & Meditation for Healing.
27. Srivastav C.M. (1999) Rudraksh Shakti Key Rahasaya (in Hindi). Manoj Publiciations, New Delhi.
28. Swami K. Satyanarayana (2003) Rudraksh Therapy. Kashi Prasad Khera Charitable Trust, Kolkatta. pp.48

29. Tapavasi Odarnath Baba & Dr. Ram Krishan Upadhyay (1997) Chamatkari Rudraksh. Randhir Prakashan, Haridwar (UP).
30. Thayyril Kumaran Krishan (1966) Ayurvediya Oshadhi Nighantu. Central Council of Ayurvedic Research, New Delhi
31. Tripathi I.D. (1982) Narahari : Raja Nighantu (Hindi-Commentary), Krishnadas Academy Publications Varanasi (UP).
32. The Wealth of India (1952) Vol. III (D-E) with Index to Vol. I & III C.S.I.R. Publication, New Delhi.
33. Tirel C (1982) Flora Non Velle Caldonia Dependences Vol. 11. p.45-47.

LEGEND

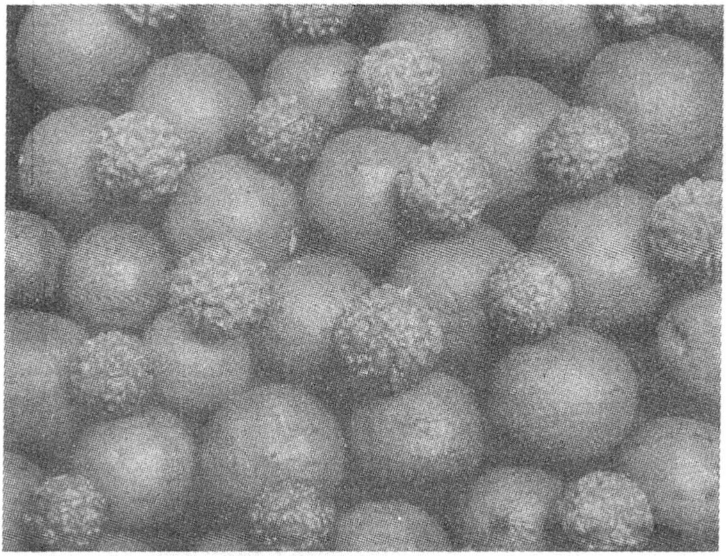

1. *Holy beads of Rudraksh alongwith their blue colour fruits*

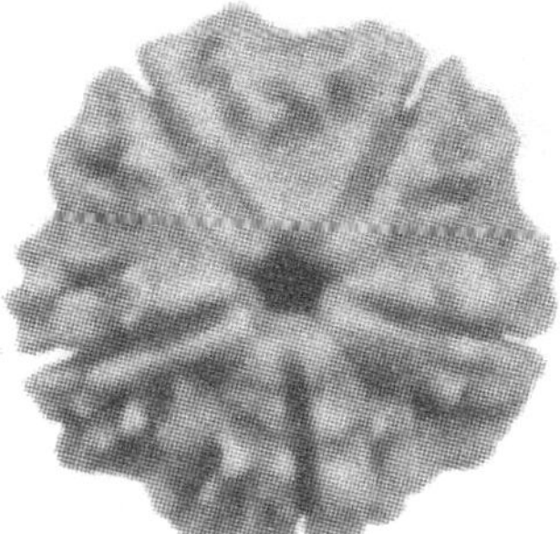

2. *Five Mukhi Rudraksh*

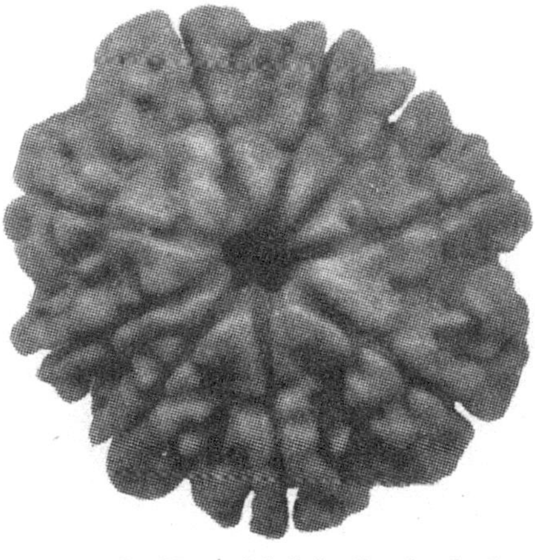

3. *Nine Mukhi Rudraksh*

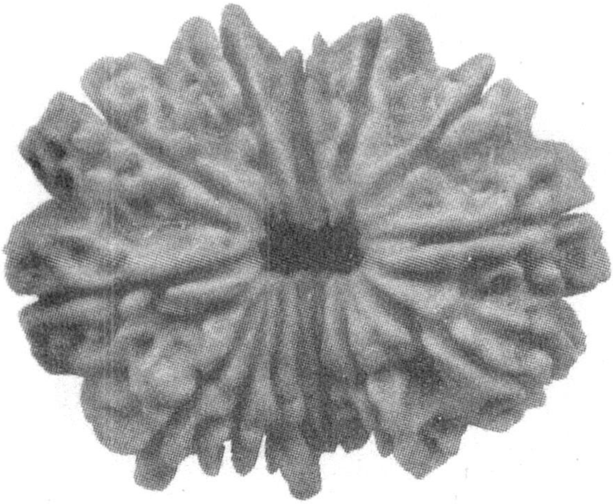

4. *Fourteen Mukhi Rudraksh*

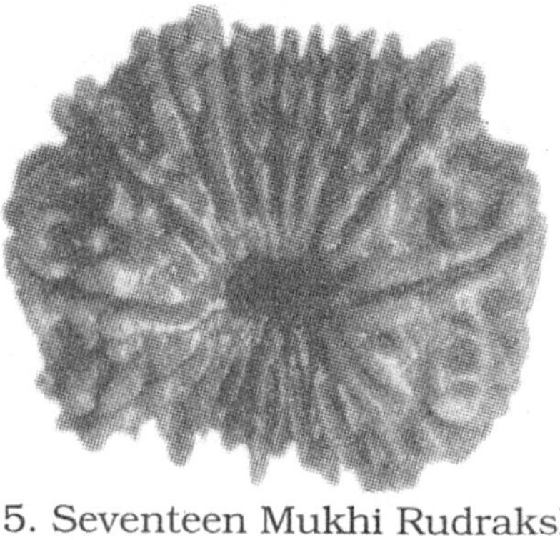

5. Seventeen Mukhi Rudraksh

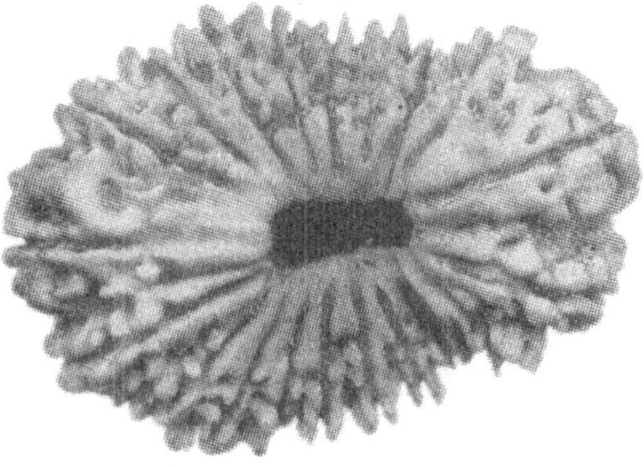

6. *Twenty One Mukhi Rudraksh*

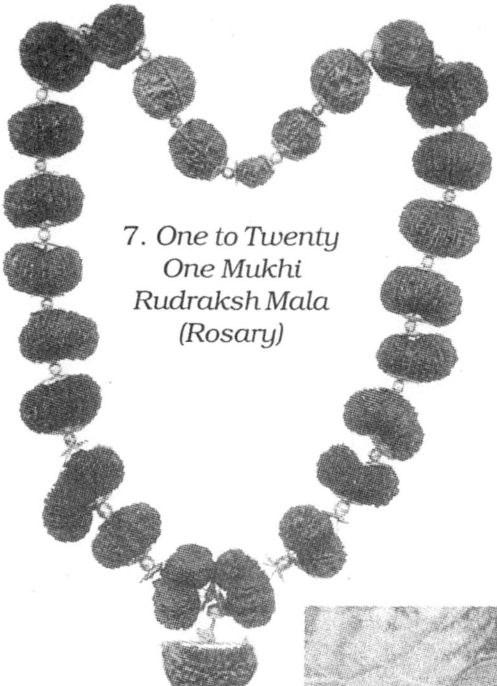

7. One to Twenty One Mukhi Rudraksh Mala (Rosary)

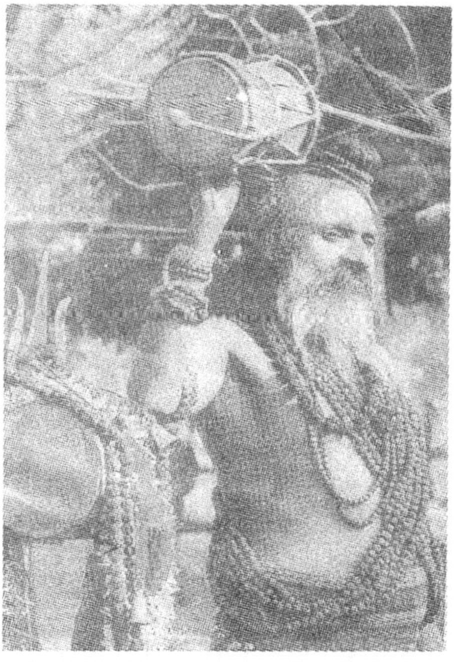

8. A Sadhu wearing Rudraksh Mala as his Spiritual Attire.

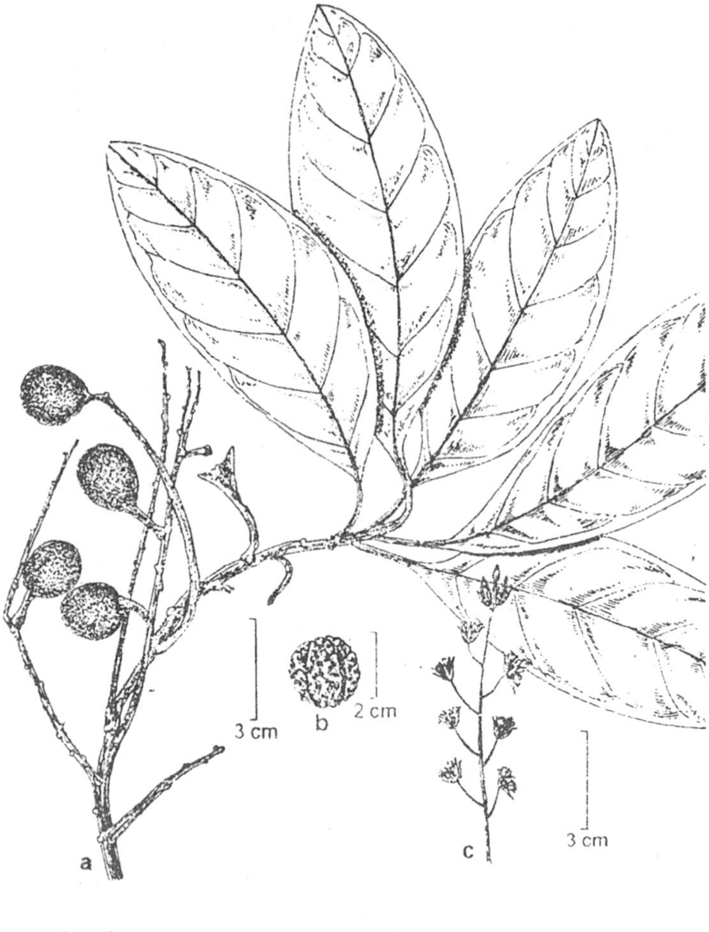

9. *Elaeocarpus ganitrus a. fruiting twig; b. nut; c. part of inflorescence.*